Cochlear Implants

Objective Measures

Cochlear Implants

Objective Measures

Edited by

HELEN E CULLINGTON BSc, MSc

House Ear Institute
Los Angeles

W
WHURR PUBLISHERS
LONDON AND PHILADELPHIA

© 2003 Whurr Publishers Ltd
First published 2003
by Whurr Publishers Ltd
19b Compton Terrace, London N1 2UN, England and
325 Chestnut Street, Philadelphia PA 19106, USA

Reprinted 2004

British Library Cataloguing in Publication Data
A catalogue record for this book is available from the British
Library.

ISBN 978-1-86156-324-8

Contents

Contributors

Rolf-Dieter Battmer
Department of Otolaryngology
Medical University
Hannover
Germany

Carolyn J Brown
Department of Speech Pathology and Audiology and
Department of Otolaryngology – Head and Neck Surgery
University of Iowa
Iowa City
Iowa
USA

Stacy L Butts
University of Miami Ear Institute
Miami
Florida
USA

Paul Carter
Cochlear Corporation
Englewood
Colorado
USA

Helen E Cullington
Care Center
House Ear Institute
Los Angeles
California
USA

Manuel Don
Department of Electrophysiology
House Ear Institute
Los Angeles
California
USA

Gail Feinman
University of Colorado School of Medicine
Denver
Colorado
USA

Jill B Firszt
Department of Otolaryngology and Communication Sciences
Medical College of Wisconsin
Milwaukee
Wisconsin
USA

Annelle V Hodges
University of Miami Ear Institute
Miami
Florida
USA

Paul R Kileny
Department of Otolaryngology
University of Michigan Health System
Ann Arbor
Michigan
USA

John E King
University of Miami Ear Institute
Miami
USA

Steve Mason
Medical Physics Department
Queen's Medical Centre
Nottingham
United Kingdom

Lucas H M Mens
Cochlear Implant Centrum Nijmegen | Sint-Michielsgestel
University Medical Center Nijmegen
The Netherlands

Curtis W Ponton
Neuroscan Labs
El Paso
Texas
USA

Jon K Shallop
Mayo Clinic
Rochester
Minnesota
USA

Bruce Tabor
Cochlear Limited
Lane Cove
New South Wales
Australia

Foreword

Twenty-five years ago acceptance of cochlear implants by hearing research professionals was not universal. Many raised concerns about safety and doubted an electrical stimulus within the cochlea of a deaf patient would provide any benefit. Over the years, patient outcome studies have shown implants to be safe and beneficial. Initially, many of the studies were based on the subjective responses of the patients. More recently, hearing professionals have developed objective measures that are helpful in the assessment and management of implant patients.

Cochlear Implants: Objective Measures is an excellent review of many of the objective measures presently available. The book provides answers to: what are objective measures, why do them and how to perform them. Advances in implant technology in external and internal hardware and software components have led to substantial improvement in post-implant performance. It is hoped that the objective measures reviewed in this book will lead to further enhancement of performance.

William M Luxford MD
House Ear Clinic
Los Angeles
October 2002

Acknowledgements

I would like to thank the following people for their help and support: Manny Don, Jill Firszt, Mark Lutman and Steve Mason. In addition I am grateful to all my colleagues at the Institute of Sound and Vibration Research, University of Southampton, and House Ear Institute, Los Angeles.

Introduction

The success of cochlear implantation is well documented and many centres are now implanting very young children and those with multiple disabilities. The need for objective measures to confirm candidacy, verify device function and set programming parameters has therefore increased.

In September 1998, the First International Symposium and Workshop on Objective Measures in Cochlear Implantation was held in Nottingham in the UK. This meeting was a tremendous success, with over 130 participants from 17 countries. This was followed by a second meeting in Lyon, France in March 2001. The attendance at these events shows the high level of interest worldwide in objective measures. In addition, objective measures now make up a significant number of the papers presented at all international cochlear implant conferences.

The authors of this book are all experienced clinicians and researchers in the field of cochlear implantation. In a multi-author book of this nature there will be inevitable repetition of information or differences in opinion. I hope that the repetition will enable readers to assimilate the facts from different perspectives, perhaps even allowing selection of topic coverage to match their background, experience and interest. Differences in opinion may intrigue readers and stimulate them to seek their own answers!

This book provides the clinician with a guide to the objective measures available in the field of cochlear implantation. All these tests are used clinically but there is also much ongoing research. As new features of devices are implemented and research breaks new ground it is likely that some areas of this book will be out of date soon after publication. I hope, though, that it will provide the reader with a sound basis to understand the applications of objective measures in cochlear implantation.

Chapter 1

Introduction to cochlear implant objective measures

Helen E Cullington, Rolf-Dieter Battmer

Contents

- What are objective measures?
- Why are objective measures important?
- How to record objective measures.
- The future of objective measures.

This chapter aims to cover some basic questions about objective measures in cochlear implantation in order to prepare the reader for the more detailed information that follows.

What are objective measures?

Audiologists are accustomed to using objective procedures such as otoacoustic emissions, the stapedial reflex, the auditory brainstem response and cortical evoked potentials to supplement behavioural data. Techniques that do not rely on patient participation are equally important in the field of cochlear implants.

Objective measures used with cochlear implants can be divided into two categories: electrical measures and electrophysiological measures. New imaging techniques are being investigated, although these are not yet used clinically.

Electrical measures

Electrical measures have been developed to evaluate the function of the implant electronics and the electrode output. Most cochlear implant devices include a telemetry system; this transmits information about the implant and electrode status to the outside (to the fitting station and/or the speech processor). This has made new electrical measures available to the clinician. The electrical measures are covered in detail in Chapters 2 and 3; the main procedures are as follows:

- troubleshooting external components such as processor, microphone, cables;
- internal implant electronics test;
- testing radio frequency (RF) coupling;
- electrode impedance telemetry;
- compliance voltage telemetry;
- electrical field imaging;
- averaged electrode voltages.

Electrical measures provide valuable information at the time of cochlear implant surgery and postoperatively, to confirm device function and to investigate the integrity of the electrode contacts.

Troubleshooting external components

Most devices now feature alarms or a display indicating that the external equipment — the processor, microphone and cables — is intact. Figure 1.1 shows the LCD display on the Nucleus® SPrint™ speech processor. The upper section of the display shows the program number, and volume and sensitivity settings. The lower section shows all the troubleshooting symbols.

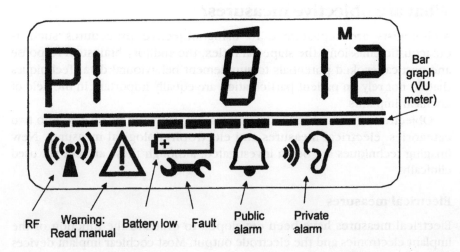

Figure 1.1. LCD display of the Nucleus® SPrint™ speech processor showing the troubleshooting symbols.

The following information is provided to the user:

- audio level meter;
- RF test;
- warning: read the manual;
- low battery;
- system fault: servicing required;
- public and private alarms to indicate low battery.

Internal implant electronics test

Most implant systems allow the clinician to check the internal implanted electronics through the fitting software, and some perform a similar check automatically every time the processor is switched on. Some devices also allow an implant test to be undertaken before the cochlear implant is even removed from its packaging, thus allowing the clinician or surgeon to be confident that the device is intact.

Testing RF coupling

All current cochlear implant systems send power and information across the skin using RF transmission. It is vital to test and optimize this RF link to avoid intermittent hearing sensations. Most systems provide clinicians and parents with a means to check the RF output, and the Advanced Bionics Corporation CLARION® system allows the RF power to be optimized for individual users.

Electrode impedance telemetry

One of the most important applications of the communication link available in new implant systems is the ability to test the electrode contacts by measuring their impedances. Very high values may indicate an open circuit, whereas very low impedances may indicate a short circuit between electrode contacts. This provides instant information about the status of the electrode array. Generally impedance measures are used very frequently after surgery: many centres will use them at every patient appointment to monitor system integrity.

It is also possible to obtain impedance and electronics test measures prior to implantation by placing the device in saline and thus performing *in vitro* measurements. However, this is generally not recommended by the manufacturers due to the increased handling of the device that is involved.

Compliance voltage telemetry

Another important electrical measure is compliance voltage telemetry; this assesses whether the implant current source is able to output the required stimulation amplitude. A current source will be out of compliance if the required current for the particular impedance exceeds the maximum supply voltage within the implant. This means that an increase in mapping current levels will no longer result in an increase in loudness for the patient.

Electrical field imaging

A new form of telemetry is the assessment of the electrical field set up within the cochlea. This is accomplished by stimulating one channel and simultaneously measuring voltages on all non-stimulated channels. Some systems use this to detect short circuits in the electrode array, in addition to assessing the longitudinal voltage gradient along the electrode array. This gradient may be related to how selectively each channel stimulates the nerve. Mens and Mulder (2001) completed some interesting investigations into the electrical field generated by the CLARION HiFocus™ electrode array, both with and without the Electrode Positioning System™.

Averaged electrode voltages

The electrical output of a device can be evaluated by recording the surface potentials at the scalp resulting from the stimulation currents of the implant. When sampled and averaged, these potentials are known as averaged electrode voltages (AEVs) or sometimes integrity testing. Using this technique, an image of stimulation pulses of one channel or a sweep of all channels can be obtained (Almqvist et al., 1993; Battmer et al., 1994). By manipulating various parameters (for example comparing bipolar, monopolar and common ground modes of stimulation) information can be obtained about the integrity of the device, and also in some cases certain cochlear pathologies can be detected (Carter, 2001). (See Appendix 1.1 of this chapter for an explanation of different stimulation modes.) Figure 1.2 shows an example of AEVs recorded in bipolar + 1 (BP+1) mode, using the Crystal Integrity Test System. The Crystal is a purpose-built integrity test system for the Nucleus cochlear implants; it is described in detail in Chapter 3. Biphasic voltage pulse responses are seen from 20 electrodes.

Electrophysiological measures

Electrophysiological measures are those that involve interaction with the human physiology. This differentiates them from purely electrical measures, which can be studied *in vitro*. Electrophysiological measures can evaluate most areas of the auditory pathways, from the early compound action potentials generated in the cochlea to the central auditory areas.

Conventional electrophysiological measures are evoked by auditory stimulation (for example the auditory brainstem response). However it is also possible to use electrical stimulation, either through the cochlear implant or

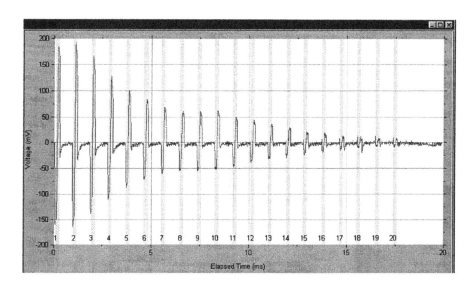

Figure 1.2. Averaged electrode voltages recorded in BP+1 mode using the Crystal Integrity Test system.

by placement of a temporary electrode at or near the cochlea. For each auditory electrophysiological measure there is a corresponding electrically evoked electrophysiological measure; therefore most areas of the auditory pathways can be evaluated.

The most commonly used electrically evoked measures are listed below, including reference to the chapter that discusses each one in detail:

- electrically evoked stapedial reflex (ESR) (Chapter 4);
- electrically evoked whole nerve/compound action potential (EAP or ECAP) (Chapter 5);
- electrically evoked auditory brainstem response (EABR) (Chapter 6);
- electrically evoked middle latency response (EMLR) (Chapter 7);
- electrically evoked cortical auditory evoked potentials (AEPs) (Chapter 7 and Chapter 8).

It is common convention to prefix the standard abbreviation for the evoked potential with an E, to indicate an electrically evoked potential. With the exception of the ECAP, which requires a near-field recording electrode, these measures can all be obtained before implant surgery using a temporary stimulation electrode placed close to the cochlea. The earlier measures (ECAP, ESR and EABR) can be recorded during the implant surgery, and all potentials can be used at any time postoperatively.

Electrically evoked stapedial reflex

The ESR has been studied for several years. It is essentially identical to the acoustically evoked reflex in all but the eliciting stimulus. An example is shown in Figure 1.3. The ESRs have been measured in the reflex decay screen of a GSI 33 immittance meter. Two stimuli were used, and the double deflections corresponding to the reflex can clearly be seen. The stimulus ranged from 188 down to 182 current units. The ESR can be recorded during and after cochlear implant surgery. In addition to providing confirmation of device and auditory system function, postoperative ESR thresholds have been shown to correlate well with behavioural comfort (C) levels in the Nucleus 22, Nucleus 24, CLARION and MED-EL devices (for example Hodges et al., 1997, 1999 and 2000; Butts et al., 2001).

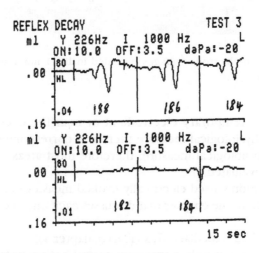

Figure 1.3. Typical electrically evoked stapedial reflexes.

Electrically evoked compound action potential

The objective measure that is perhaps the topic of the most research projects at the moment is the ECAP. This is also known as the electrically evoked whole nerve action potential (EAP). The ECAP is called Neural Response Telemetry (NRT™) when measured using the Nucleus 24 device, and when using the CLARION CII device it is called Neural Response Imaging (NRI). Figure 1.4 shows an example of NRT responses obtained at several different stimulation levels. The response consists of a negative deflection (N1) with a latency of around 0.3 ms, and a positive peak (P1) at around 0.6 ms. The ECAP measurement is the electrical equivalent of electrocochleography. The intracochlear electrodes of the cochlear implant device are used both for

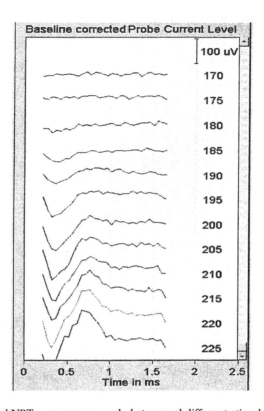

Figure 1.4. Typical NRT responses recorded at several different stimulation levels.

stimulation and recording of the response, with no additional evoked potentials equipment required. Due to the proximity of the recording electrode to the neural elements, the ECAP is a large amplitude response, and is resilient to movement artefacts. This makes it ideal for measurement in children, who do not need to be sedated or remain still. From a survey at the end of the year 2000, Cochlear Ltd estimated that over 250 clinics worldwide were using NRT clinically, with more than 2,000 documented cases; this number is expected to be much higher now (Cafarelli Dees, personal communication).

A disadvantage of measuring the ECAP, however, is that the recording site is very close to the stimulation, thus generating a very large stimulus artefact. Several methods have been proposed to eliminate this artefact; these are discussed in detail in Chapter 5.

The ECAP can be recorded during or after cochlear implant surgery; it is used to confirm response to electrical stimulation, monitor changes over time, and assist with setting programming levels. There is also hope that it may in future assist in the selection of programming strategy, although there is little conclusive evidence of this so far.

Electrically evoked auditory brainstem response

The EABR has a role to play at all stages of cochlear implantation. It can be recorded before implantation, using electrical stimulation at the promontory or round window, and is often recorded both intraoperatively and postoperatively.

In the past, promontory stimulation EABR (prom-EABR) was used quite frequently during assessment of candidacy for cochlear implantation, in order to confirm auditory sensation with electrical stimulation. In some cases, the results were used to select which ear to implant (for example, Mason et al., 1997). However, recent research has questioned the value of this procedure as many children with absent prom-EABRs still receive significant benefit from a cochlear implant (Nikolopoulos et al., 2000). Figure 1.5 shows EABR responses recorded from different stimulation sites, compared with the acoustic ABR.

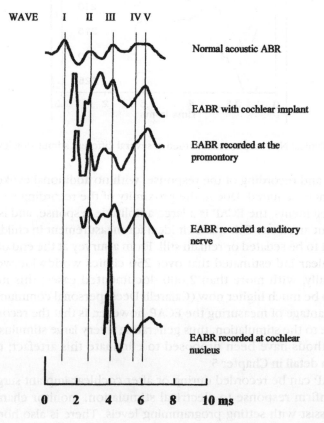

Figure 1.5. Electrically evoked auditory brainstem responses recorded from different stimulation sites, compared with the acoustic ABR (adapted from Frohne, 2000).

Electrically evoked auditory brainstem response thresholds are typically higher than behavioural threshold (T) levels, although the exact difference has varied across studies. They can provide assistance with mapping. Gallégo et al. (1998) showed a relationship between latency measures of the EABR and performance with the cochlear implant, although other researchers do not replicate this. Abbas and Brown (1991) were unable to demonstrate a relation between the amplitude input/output function of the EABR and performance. Researchers in Japan (Kubo et al., 2001) found that the EABR input/output function was only correlated with performance at one month after implantation, and not at any later times. They concluded that as the amplitude growth function reflects the number of remaining spiral ganglion cells in the inner ear, a large number of surviving cells is only advantageous for initial performance. However these studies varied in their stimuli, recording parameters, and times of measurement, so it is not possible to directly compare findings and further research is required. Certainly there are many factors that affect performance with a cochlear implant, and it is unlikely that measures of lower brainstem function, as reflected by the EABR, would fully explain or predict performance.

Electrically evoked auditory brainstem response measurements are also of great importance during auditory brainstem implant (ABI) surgery. With the help of EABR recordings the correct placement of the ABI electrode on the cochlear nucleus can be confirmed and possible non-auditory side effects can be minimized.

Electrically evoked middle latency response and cortical auditory evoked potentials

There is a very wide range in performance of cochlear implant users, even among those with similar characteristics – for example aetiology, device and processing strategy. It is known that speech recognition requires both the peripheral and central auditory systems; therefore there has been much interest in studying electrically evoked later latency auditory potentials, in order to attempt to explain performance characteristics.

The electrically evoked middle latency response (EMLR) is similar in appearance to the acoustic MLR (Firszt, 1998). Figure 1.6 shows the response recorded from a CLARION cochlear implant user. There is a clear negative deflection (Na) and a later positive peak (Pa). Research has shown good correlation between EMLR thresholds and behavioural T levels (for example Firszt, 1998). Response parameters also show a relation to speech under-standing scores (such as Groenen et al., 2000).

The late latency auditory evoked potentials are believed to arise from the thalamus and auditory cortex. The electrically evoked cortical AEPs that have been most studied are the N1, P2, P300 and MMN (mismatch negativity)

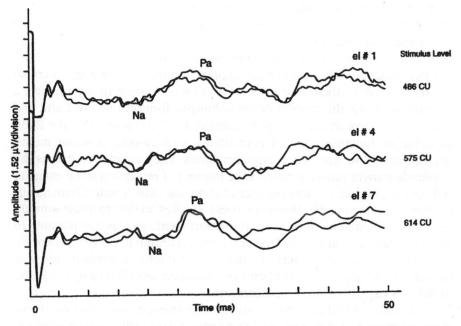

Figure 1.6. Electrically evoked middle latency response from a CLARION cochlear implant user, following stimulation on three electrodes (adapted from Firszt, 1998).

responses. Research has shown that cortical evoked activity can reliably be obtained from cochlear implant users, with the responses being similar to those obtained from normally hearing subjects. Figure 1.7 shows cortical AEPs recorded from an adult cochlear implant user; the P1, N1 and P2 features can clearly be seen, in addition to the massive stimulus artefact.

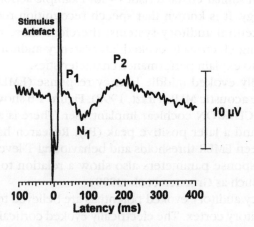

Figure 1.7. Electrically evoked cortical AEPs from an adult cochlear implant user.

Auditory evoked potentials can be divided into those that are exogenous (characteristics are determined by external stimuli) or endogenous (influenced by internal cognitive processes). However this classification is often blurred in the case of the late latency potentials. Endogenous potentials can be known as event-related potentials. Perhaps the most well-known event-related potential is the MMN. This uses an oddball stimulus paradigm, consisting of a frequently repeated stimulus, randomly interspersed with an infrequently repeated deviant stimulus. Many acoustic differences can be used to evoke the MMN, including frequency, duration, intensity, and more complex speech sounds. The presence of the MMN response therefore reflects the ability to discriminate between sounds. Kraus et al. (1993) analysed the MMN in cochlear implant users and found that those with better speech perception had more robust MMNs.

Ponton and his colleagues have used cortical AEPs to investigate the effects of deafness and cochlear implant use on the maturation of the central nervous system (for example, Ponton et al., 2000). This opens up some exciting avenues for research. Ponton suggests that cortical evoked responses such as the MMN may be used to monitor an implant user's progress, and provide individualized targeted rehabilitation programmes. The responses may also be able to predict an individual's potential for performance (Ponton, 2001), although much further research is required in this area.

The cortical AEPs have the advantage that their longer latency makes the recording epoch further from the contaminating stimulus artefact; an additional benefit is that they can be evoked by speech and other complex sounds. However the disadvantage is that they are strongly influenced by age, sleep stage and attention, therefore making them more problematic in young children.

It is possible to record the later potentials using promontory stimulation before cochlear implant surgery in cooperative awake adults and adolescents (Deggouj et al., 2001). However promontory stimulation requires sedation or anaesthetic in young children, therefore adversely affecting the responses. The responses can be recorded at any stage postoperatively, but in children it is often more difficult to maintain the correct state of arousal.

Imaging techniques

Two new techniques are currently under investigation: positron emission tomography (PET) and functional magnetic resonance imaging (fMRI). These methods allow the perfusion of the central auditory system to be visualized after acoustic or electrical stimulation. Magnetic resonance imaging is generally contraindicated in cochlear implant patients, although it can be performed under controlled conditions. Figure 1.8 shows a PET scan of the brain both with and without electrical stimulation through a cochlear

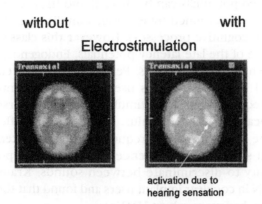

activation due to
hearing sensation

Figure 1.8. PET scan of the brain both with and without electrical stimulation through a cochlear implant (adapted from Lesinski-Schiedat, 2000).

implant. The cortical activation resulting from hearing sensation with electrical stimulation is visualized by comparing the transaxial planes with and without electrical stimulation.

This book aims to be a practical handbook for clinicians, and therefore the imaging techniques are beyond its scope. They are currently research tools and require considerable further study before they can be applied clinically. The reader is invited to consult the references listed at the end of this chapter for further information (Naito et al., 1995; Okazawa et al., 1996; Schmid et al., 1998).

Why are objective measures important?

Objective measures are used in cochlear implantation for the following main reasons:

- confirmation of candidacy;
- verification of device and auditory system function;
- setting programming parameters;
- research into auditory system mechanics.

Table 1.1 summarizes the main functions of objective measures used in cochlear implantation.

Confirmation of candidacy

Standard audiological objective measures are vital in the process of assessing candidacy for cochlear implantation. They aim to evaluate the integrity of the

Table 1.1. Overview of the main functions of objective measures used in cochlear implantation

Test	Can assess candidacy preimplant	Assesses implant function	Assesses auditory system function	Assists with setting mapping levels	Predicts or evaluates performance
Telemetry		✓			
Averaged electrode voltages (AEV)		✓			
Electrically evoked stapedial reflex (ESR)			✓	✓	
Electrically evoked compound action potential (ECAP)			✓	✓	
Electrically evoked auditory brainstem response (EABR)	✓		✓	✓	✓
Electrically evoked middle latency (EMLR) and cortical AEPs	✓		✓	✓	✓
Electrically evoked event-related potentials (ERP)	✓		✓	✓	✓

auditory pathways and verify the extent and site of the hearing loss. Electrophysiological techniques are very well covered in many audiology texts and are outside the remit of this book.

However, there has been much interest in whether or not electrically evoked auditory potentials (particularly evoked potentials recorded preoperatively) could be used to predict postimplant performance with a cochlear implant. It was thought that if one could estimate the degree of neural survival a patient had prior to surgery it might allow a more informed decision regarding cochlear implantation, or assist in selection of the better ear to implant. In general though, results with preimplant electrical recordings have been quite variable and inconclusive.

Verification of device and auditory system function

Cochlear implant devices are extremely reliable. Over 4,000 recipients have been implanted for more than a year now with the strengthened Nucleus CI24 cochlear implant system. The Cumulative Survival Percentage (CSP) at one year is 99.9% for adults and 99.3% for children (*Nucleus Reliability Update,* Issue 4, 2001). However the possibility of failure always exists. The total number of cochlear implant recipients worldwide now exceeds 40,000 (*Nucleus Report,* October 2001). This large and ever increasing number of devices means that all centres will eventually be faced with a device failure.

An implant failure can occur for a variety of reasons, for instance: electronic circuit failures, mechanical failures of the implant casing, or breakage of the electrode array. These faults may occur spontaneously, or as a result of trauma to the device. Whenever there is suspicion of a device failure, immediate action must be taken as it will be an anxious time for the patient and his or her family. Electrical measures are vital in these situations. Impedance testing and electrical field imaging will provide valuable information, however the preferred test is usually measurement of averaged electrode voltages (AEVs). Intermittent system faults are usually the most difficult to detect and manage, and often require several tests.

In addition to device failure, the patient's interaction with the device must also be considered. The reason for a sudden loss of hearing through the implant could be a preoperatively undetected or a later acquired disease of the peripheral or central auditory pathways. In this case, electrophysiological techniques can be used, for example assessing the ECAP or EABR.

Faults with the external equipment are much more common, but equally important to detect and remedy. The cables are the weakest link in the chain of external components; these need to be replaced every few months, or even more frequently for active young children.

Setting programming parameters

Effective programming is necessary for maximum benefit from cochlear implants. The process of setting the programming parameters is referred to as mapping, programming or tuning. Programming multichannel cochlear implants requires that the patient make a series of judgements regarding perception of the stimuli being presented through the implant. The implant user should confirm that the stimulation being received on each stimulation site is auditory. If the patient is able to specify that a particular electrode produces an odd sensation, accommodations can be made by the programmer to alleviate the problem.

The patient must then provide a minimum response level. This is the current level required to produce a 'just audible' percept to the listener. Depending on the device, the minimal stimulation level may be set at a 100% detection rate, 50% detection rate, or a level slightly below the just audible percept. Setting the minimal level too high may have negative effects, such as increasing the level of background noise or producing an audible hum in the processor. Setting the minimal level too low may result in the inability to hear certain soft sounds. This threshold of electrical stimulation is known as the T level.

Each device also requires the establishment of a maximum stimulation level. The maximum level is used in the stimulation algorithm to prevent uncomfortably loud sound from reaching the listener. If maximum stimulation levels are set too low, the dynamic range would be artificially reduced, resulting in speech that is overall too soft, with little variation in intensity. If maximum stimulation levels are set too high, speech can become distorted, and certain loud sounds may be uncomfortable. The maximum stimulation level is usually called the comfort level (C level) or the most comfortable level (MCL or M level).

Finally, if speech is to sound as smooth and natural as possible, the maximum stimulation levels should be of approximately equal loudness across the array. If the patient uses the same criteria to judge the maximum level for each electrode, the loudness should be balanced. If not, the quality of speech may be choppy, tinny, or hollow.

These judgements require that the listener understand concepts such as loud, most comfortable loudness, maximum comfortable loudness, uncomfortable loudness, and equal loudness. He or she must also be able to convey the judgements to the programmer. In order to set the threshold levels, behavioural and observational audiometric techniques (for example visual reinforcement audiometry and conditioned play audiometry) can be used in some children with reasonable accuracy. The maximum comfortable stimulation levels should be estimated cautiously by observing the child's behaviour when the stimuli are presented. In all cases, it is best to avoid reaching stimulation levels that result in an uncomfortably loud level. If this occurs, the child may temporarily stop participating in the programming session, which delays setting of the external speech processor. Loudness judgements can be difficult even for cooperative adult patients. Young children, especially those deafened prelingually, often do not have the necessary language base or auditory experience to report loudness; however the concepts can be taught as the children use their implant and gain experience over time.

Many countries now implement a neonatal hearing screening programme; the benefit of early identification is that appropriate intervention can be commenced immediately. Studies have shown that children who receive amplification prior to 6–12 months of age have better long-term outcomes in terms of speech and language development than children who receive the same intervention at a later date (Yoshinaga-Itano et al., 1998; Moeller, 2000). Many professionals view cochlear implantation as the treatment of choice for individuals with profound, bilateral sensorineural hearing loss. As such, both parents and professionals working with young, congenitally hearing-impaired children feel a need to expedite the cochlear implant surgery.

Programming a child's cochlear implant can require numerous return visits to develop a map that produces high sound quality. The benefit of early implantation is minimized if programming levels are grossly inaccurate. Older children may have a short attention span, thus limiting the amount of information available during one session. In addition, it may be extremely difficult to obtain reliable behavioural measures from individuals with multiple developmental delays. For these reasons, it is vital that a battery of objective measures be available to assist with setting the speech processor, in conjunction with behavioural measures.

The current generation of cochlear implant systems features a choice of many programming parameters and strategies. Although an adult may be able to evaluate two or three strategies and select their preference; this is usually not possible for children. Research is therefore focusing on using objective measures to assist in the selection of the optimum parameters for individual patients. This research has mainly used the ECAP, and although early results are promising, no definite predictions are available.

Research into auditory system mechanics

The ability to measure auditory potentials evoked by electrical stimulation enables research into the mechanics of the auditory system. For example, it is possible to use electrophysiological techniques to investigate the effects of long periods of auditory deprivation and/or congenital hearing loss on the auditory system, as discussed earlier.

How to record objective measures

Detailed procedures for obtaining objective measures in cochlear implant patients will be covered in later chapters. However one significant difficulty with obtaining all electrically evoked electrophysiological measures is the presence of artefact contaminating the neural potential of interest. This is usually from the electrical stimulus, but can also be as a result of the RF transmission of power and data across the skin used by all current cochlear implant systems. Methods of artefact reduction are covered in the following chapters, especially in Chapter 8.

The future of objective measures

It seems likely that the age of implantation will drop even further in the future, with implantation during the first year of life becoming routine. In order for this to occur, much more reliance will have to be placed on objective measures, for the diagnostic evaluation of hearing thresholds and amplification benefit, and in the subsequent programming of the cochlear implant device. The ultimate aim would be accurate diagnosis and confirmation of hearing levels near to birth, with appropriate programming of the cochlear implant occurring at the time of initial stimulation. The following topics are a small selection of current research that has caught the eye of the authors.

Several alternative techniques to estimate infants' hearing thresholds are currently being assessed. One such method involves recording the steady state evoked potential (SSEP). This has the advantages of being frequency specific, using automatic response detection criteria, and being recordable at louder levels than current ABR equipment allows. Results indicate that the SSEP is able to accurately assess hearing thresholds (Stapells et al., 1984) and has a role in assessing the hearing of infants and young children before implantation (Firszt et al., 2001). In addition, the electrically evoked SSEP is currently being researched and may prove to be a useful tool (Brown and Abbas, personal communication).

Another less used electrophysiological response is the sympathetic skin response (SSR). This is a test of function of a polysynaptic reflex having sweat glands as effectors. The reflex is coordinated in the posterior hypothalamus or upper brainstem reticular formation (Arunodaya and Taly, 1995). A recent study has shown strong correlation between the SSR threshold and the threshold to electrical stimulation in cochlear implant patients (Péréon et al., 2001). It is hoped that research into this technique will continue.

If children are to be implanted at a very young age, in addition to the need for accurate hearing threshold information, objective testing of their speech discrimination abilities is required both before and after implantation. A behavioural technique called visual habituation (VH) procedure has been studied in normally hearing, deaf and cochlear implanted infants. It has shown potential as a technique to assess an infant's ability to detect speech contrasts and to evaluate their audiovisual speech perception skills (Houston et al., 2001). This would be a great leap forward if it became possible to evaluate speech perception ability in infants who previously could only provide hearing sensitivity results. In addition to evaluating the infant's benefit from amplification before implantation, the test would be ideally suited to assess the implanted infant, in order to target rehabilitation at areas where speech perception seems poorer.

It is now recognized that the interface between cochlear implant electrodes and the nerve fibres is in part responsible for the variability in speech perception results (Houben et al., 2001). As such this has become a focus for research. By studying ECAPs in implanted guinea pigs, Houben and colleagues demonstrated that the characteristics of the potentials varied depending upon the proximity to the modiolus. This analysis could be applied to determine the electrode positioning in human cochlear implant subjects. The electrode tissue interface has also been studied using electro-chemical impedance spectroscopy (Duan et al., 2001).

Middlebrooks and colleagues are researching cortical activation evoked by cochlear implants, using both animal models (Bierer and Middlebrooks, 2001) and artificial neural networks (Middlebrooks and Bierer, 2001). Further animal and computational modelling work is investigating the ECAP response (for example Miller et al., 1999; Lai and Dillier, 2000; Cartee et al., 2001).

One interesting approach to measurement of the electrically evoked stapedial reflex was suggested by Almqvist et al. (2000). They studied the ESR intraoperatively using an EMG needle electrode to record the response. This technique was very successful. Perhaps it would be possible for future cochlear implant devices to include an EMG electrode that is implanted into the stapedius muscle, and appropriate measurement software into their fitting software. The electrically evoked stapedial reflex could then be recorded easily at any time postoperatively, without the need for a quiet patient and an immittance meter.

We hope that research will continue in these exciting areas, providing additional objective measures to assist in the programming of a young child's cochlear implant. It has been shown that early intervention improves subsequent outcomes for the hearing-impaired child and, in the case of cochlear implantation, it is vital that clinicians can be confident that the device is set optimally for the child. Perhaps we are researching ourselves out of jobs, if objective measures become so advanced that the whole programming procedure is performed automatically! We can only wait and see what the future holds.

Acknowledgements

The authors acknowledge the substantial contribution that Carolyn Brown and Annelle Hodges made to this chapter.

References

Abbas PJ, Brown CJ (1991) Electrically evoked auditory brainstem response: growth of response with current level. Hear Res 51: 123-38.

Almqvist B, Harris H, Jonsson K-E (1993) The stimulogram. In Advances in Cochlear Implants. Proc 3rd Int Cochlear Implant Conference, Innsbruck, pp. 33-6.

Almqvist B, Harris S, Shallop JK (2000) Objective intraoperative method to record averaged electromyographic stapedius muscle reflexes in cochlear implant patients. Audiology 39: 146-52.

Arunodaya GR, Taly AB (1995) Sympathetic skin response: a decade later. J Neurol Sci 129: 81-9.

Battmer RD, Gnadeberg D, Lehnhardt E, Lenarz T (1994) An integrity test for the Nucleus Mini 22 Cochlear Implant System. Eur Arch Otorhinolaryngol 251: 205-9.

Bierer JA, Middlebrooks JC (2001) Auditory cortical images of cochlear-implant stimuli: dependence on electrode configuration. J Neurophysiol (in press).

Butts SL, Hodges AV, Balkany TJ, King JE, Bricker KK, Lingvai JR (2001) Stapedial reflexes in MED-EL cochlear implant users. Presented at the CI 2001, VIth Biennial Conference on Cochlear Implants in Children, Los Angeles, CA, USA.

Cartee LA, Finley CC, Wilson BS (2001) A model of the intracochlear evoked potential. Presented at Conference on Implantable Auditory Prostheses, Pacific Grove CA, USA.

Carter P (2001) The use of surface potential testing for diagnosing cochlear implant electrode faults and cochlear pathologies. Presented at 2nd International Symposium and Workshop on Objective Measures in Cochlear Implantation, Lyon, France.

Deggouj N, de Tourtchaninoff M, Wang J, Delinte A, Kasti M, Gersdorff M (2001) Prognostic value of late auditory potentials evoked by electric promontory stimulation in profoundly deaf subjects candidate for cochlear implantation. Presented at 2nd International Symposium and Workshop on Objective Measures in Cochlear Implantation, Lyon, France.

Duan YY, Tykocinski M, Cowan R (2001) An electrochemical impedance spectroscopy (EIS) study of high surface area cochlear electrodes during the post-implantation period. Presented at Conference on Implantable Auditory Prostheses, Pacific Grove CA, USA.

Firszt JB (1998) Electrically evoked auditory potentials recorded at three levels of the auditory pathway from multichannel cochlear implant subjects: characterization and comparison to behavioral levels. Doctoral dissertation, University of Illinois, Champaign-Urbana.

Firszt JB, Wackym PA, Gaggl W (2001) The estimation of auditory sensitivity in cochlear implant candidates using steady-state evoked potentials. Presented at Conference on Implantable Auditory Prostheses, Pacific Grove CA, USA.

Frohne C (2000) Ableitung von elektrisch evozierten Potentialen des auditorischen Systems. Dissertation an der Medizinischen Hochschule Hannover, Germany.

Gallégo S, Frachet B, Micheyl C, Truy E, Collet L (1998) Cochlear implant performance and electrically-evoked auditory brain-stem response characteristics. Electroencephalogr Clin Neurophysiol 108: 521-5.

Groenen P, Makhdoum M, Snik A, Van den Broek P (2000) Auditory middle latency responses and speech perception in cochlear implant users. In Waltzman S, Cohen N (eds) Cochlear implants. New York: Thieme Medical Publishers, pp. 134-5.

Hodges AV, Balkany TJ, Ruth RA, Lambert PR, Dolan-Ash MS, Schloffman JJ (1997) Electrical middle ear muscle reflex: use in cochlear implant programming. Otolaryngol Head Neck Surg 117: 255-61.

Hodges AV, Butts SL, Dolan-Ash MS, Balkany TJ (1999) Using electrically evoked auditory reflex thresholds to fit the CLARION cochlear implant. Ann Otol Rhinol Laryngol 108: 64-8.

Hodges AV, Butts SL, King JE, Balkany TJ (2000) Electrically elicited stapedial reflexes in Nucleus 24 cochlear implant users. Presented at CI 2000, VI International Conference on Cochlear Implants, Miami FL, USA.

Houben V, Van Immerseel L, Peeters S (2001) Comparing stimulation strategies and electrode contact positions with electrically evoked compound action potentials. Presented at Conference on Implantable Auditory Prostheses, Pacific Grove CA, USA.

Houston DM, Pisoni DB, Iler Kirk K, Ying EA, Miyamoto RT (2001) Infant speech perception following cochlear implantation: a new method for investigation. Presented at Conference on Implantable Auditory Prostheses, Pacific Grove CA, USA.

Kraus N, Micco AG, Koch DB, McGee T, Carrell T, Sharma A, Wiet RJ, Weingarten CZ (1993) The mismatch negativity cortical evoked potential elicited by speech in cochlear-implant users. Hear Res 65: 118-24.

Kubo T, Yamamoto K, Iwaki T, Matsukawa M, Doi K, Tamura M (2001) Significance of auditory evoked responses (EABR and P300) in cochlear implant subjects. Acta Otolaryngol 121(2): 257-61.

Lai WK, Dillier N (2000) A simple two-component model of the electrically evoked compound action potential in the human cochlea. Audiol Neurotol 5: 333-45.

Lesinski-Schiedat A (2000) Untersuchung zur optimalen Elektrodenposition bei Cochlea-Implantat-Patienten. Habilitationsschrift an der Medizinischen Hochschule Hannover, Germany.

Mason SM, O'Donoghue GM, Gibbin KP, Garnham CW, Jowett CA (1997) Perioperative electrical auditory brainstem response in candidates for pediatric cochlear implantation. Am J Otol 18: 466-71.

Mens LHM, Mulder JJS (2001) Telemetry of intracochlear electrode voltages (IEVs) in users of the CLARION system. Presented at 2nd International Symposium and Workshop on Objective Measures in Cochlear Implantation, Lyon, France.

Middlebrooks JC, Bierer JA (2001) Auditory cortical images of cochlear-implant stimuli: coding of stimulus channel and current level. J Neurophysiol (in press).

Miller CA, Abbas PJ, Rubinstein JT (1999) An empirically based model of the electrically evoked compound action potential. Hear Res 135: 1-18.

Moeller M (2000) Early intervention and language development in children who are deaf and hard of hearing. Pediatrics 106(3), e43.

Naito Y, Okazawa H, Honjo I, Hirano S, Takahashi H, Shiomi Y, Hoji W, Kawano M, Ishizu K, Yonekura Y (1995) Cortical activation with sound stimulation in cochlear implant users demonstrated by positron emission tomography. Cogn Brain Res 2: 207-14.

Nikolopoulos TP, Mason SM, Gibbin KP, O'Donoghue GM (2000) The prognostic value of promontory electric auditory brainstem response in pediatric cochlear implantation. Ear Hear 21: 236-41.

Okazawa H, Naito Y, Yonekura Y, Sadato N, Hirano S, Nishizawa S, Magata Y, Ishizu K, Tamaki N, Honjo I, Konishi J (1996) Cochlear implant efficiency in pre- and post-lingually deaf subjects. Brain 119(4): 1297-306.

Péréon Y, Laplaud D, Nguyen The Fich S, Radafy E (2001) A new application for the sympathetic skin response: the evaluation of auditory thresholds in cochlear implant patients. Clin Neurophysiol 112: 314-18.

Ponton CW (2001) The application of electrophysiological indices in training and rehabilitation programs for cochlear implant users. Presented at 2nd International Symposium and Workshop on Objective Measures in Cochlear Implantation, Lyon, France.

Ponton CW, Don M, Eggermont JJ, Waring MD, Kwong B, Cunningham J, Trautwein P (2000) Maturation of the mismatch negativity: effects of profound deafness and cochlear implant use. Audiol Neurootol 5: 167-85.

Schmid N, Tschopp K, Schillinger C, Bilecen D, Scheffler K, Seelig J (1998) Visualisierung zentral-auditiver Prozesse mit funktioneller Magnetresonanztomographie. Laryngorhinootologie 77: 328-31.

Stapells DR, Linden D, Suffield JB, Hamel G, Picton TW (1984) Human auditory steady state potentials. Ear Hear 5(2): 105-13.

Yoshinaga-Itano C, Sedley A, Coulter D, Mehl A (1998) Language of early- and later-identified children with hearing loss. Pediatrics 102: 1161-71.

Appendix 1.1

Several authors in this book refer to different cochlear implant stimulation modes. This describes the assumed pattern of current flow within the

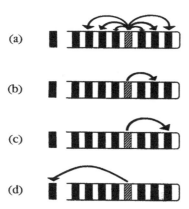

Figure 1.9. Four stimulation modes: (a) common ground; (b) bipolar + 1; (c) bipolar + 2; (d) monopolar.

cochlea. Figure 1.9 shows common ground (CG), bipolar + 1 (BP+1), bipolar + 2 (BP+2) and monopolar stimulation. In CG mode, an active electrode is selected and all other electrodes are connected together to form the indifferent electrode. In BP+1 mode, the indifferent electrode is the next but one adjacent electrode to the active. For higher bipolar modes, the indifferent electrode is moved progressively further from the active; for example in BP+2 mode the indifferent electrode is three electrodes away. In monopolar mode, the active electrode is referenced to an extra-cochlear electrode contact; this can be a ball electrode placed in the temporalis muscle, or an electrode contact on the implant casing.

CHAPTER 2

Telemetry: features and applications

LUCAS H M MENS

Contents

- Introduction.
- Troubleshooting common technical failures.
- Testing and optimizing the RF coupling.
- Telemetry of electrode impedances.
- Compliance voltage telemetry.
- Assessing the distribution of the electrical field.
- A look into the future.

Introduction

Cochlear implant systems increasingly provide information about the functioning of the internal device through telemetry. The term 'telemetry' describes the measurement and transmission of data from a remote source to a receiving station for recording and analysis. All currently produced cochlear implant systems rely on a radio frequency (RF) link through the skin to send data to the implant, as well as to receive data from the implant. Obtaining data from the implant is sometimes called 'back telemetry', because the speech processor performs 'forward telemetry' by measuring sound and sending the encoded signal to the internal device. However, for simplicity we will reserve the term 'telemetry' for the process of obtaining data from the RF link and the implant. Telemetric measures encompass the technical integrity of the RF link and the implant, the effectiveness of the electrode–tissue interface and even aspects of the evoked neural activity.

Telemetry became available in some implant systems in the early 1990s, primarily to check the integrity of the implanted electronics and the electrode array. Some five years later the first physiological response was recorded via telemetry in a clinical implant. The evoked compound action potential of the auditory nerve was measured by scanning voltages on non-stimulated electrodes in the first few milliseconds after presentation of a short pulse. The exciting possibility that peripheral excitability can be assessed in a relatively easy, non-invasive way has led to a host of studies and clinical applications. This is covered in Chapter 5. It is hoped that telemetry will provide access to other aspects of the physiological responses evoked by electrical stimulation in the near future. Without doubt, it will increasingly contribute to basic troubleshooting and integrity checking of external and internal components, thus supporting users, parents and clinicians alike.

Telemetry circuits have been designed in two ways. Some implants possess a telemetry coil separate from the receiver coil, allowing telemetry to be performed simultaneously with normal use. Other systems need to be run in a telemetry mode accessible through the clinical interface hardware. In the latter case, telemetry is performed by modulating the behaviour of the receiver coil, which affects the coupling to the transmitter coil detectable by the processor. Table 2.1 summarizes the telemetry features in the implant systems that are currently produced by three companies. Unfortunately, a fourth manufacturer, MXM, was unable to provide the relevant data.

This chapter reviews telemetry as a tool to check the integrity and effectiveness of the chain of components from processor to electrode array in setting up an electrical field capable of stimulating the auditory nerve. The chain of components involves external parts attached to the processor, the RF link, the internal receiver/stimulator, the electrode leads and electrode contacts. In addition, the electrical field inside the cochlea itself can be examined using telemetry.

Troubleshooting common technical failures

Probably the most common reason for non-stimulation during everyday use is a broken microphone cable or transmitter cable. Replacing these cables in many cases solves the problem in a single step and advanced testing procedures may seem unnecessary. However, if the failure is intermittent, it may be more difficult for the user. A broken cable may not be discernible from other defects such as unreliable battery contacts or a weak RF link due to misalignment of the transmitter and receiver coil. Even these comparatively simple problems often cause anxiety because an implant failure is feared. In the ideal case, the user (or parent) would be able to enter a diagnostic mode in which the continuous integrity of the main components including the microphone, cables and transmitter is time-stamped and logged in the speech processor over a period of time for comprehensive analysis afterwards. This would allow detection of intermittent problems, obviously at the cost of increased complexity of the system.

Table 2.1. Summary of telemetry features in three implant systems

The information below represents the features within the currently produced cochlear implants for each company. These are as follows:

Advanced Bionics Corporation, USA: CLARION CII cochlear implant and Platinum Sound Processor™; SCLIN2000 fitting software, Clinical Programming Interface

Cochlear Limited, Australia: Nucleus® 24 Contour™ cochlear implant and SPrint™ processor, WinDPS fitting software, Programming Control Interface

MED-EL, Austria: COMBI 40+ cochlear implant and TEMPO+ processor; CI.STUDIO+ fitting software, Diagnostic Interface Box

	CLARION	Nucleus	MED-EL
User alarms (light or audible)	Yes	Yes	Yes
Battery low	Yes	Yes	Yes
Corrupted speech processor	Yes	Yes	Yes
Cable failure	Yes	Yes	Yes
RF link not established	Yes	Yes	No
Microphone output detector	Yes	Yes	Yes
Microphone check by earphones	Yes	Yes	No
Mode of telemetry	Concurrent[1]	Switched[2]	Switched[3]
Strength of RF coupling test	Yes[4]	No[5]	Yes
Implant electronics self test when turned on	Yes	Yes	No
Implant electronics test by clinician	Yes	Yes	Yes[6]
Compliance telemetry	No	Yes[7]	Yes[8]
Impedance telemetry	Yes[9]	Yes[10]	Yes[9,11,12,13]
Electrical field telemetry	Experimental	No	Yes
Evoked response telemetry	Experimental	Yes[14]	No

1 Telemetry through a second RF link separate from the primary used for power and speech data. Primary signal carrier at 49 MHz, secondary at 10.7 MHz.
2 Telemetry through modulation of the receiver circuit. Primary signal carrier at 5 MHz.
3 As 2. Primary signal carrier at 10 MHz.
4 Also continuous RF power optimization during normal use.
5 Hardware supported; not yet available to clinician.
6 Including part of the output circuit using an on-board resistor.
7 Based on implant supply voltage.
8 Calculated on previously measured impedances.
9 Monopolar coupling.
10 Monopolar and common ground coupling.
11 Bipolar combinations of electrodes.
12 Extended analysis of short circuited electrodes.
13 Estimation of the ground electrode impedance.
14 Not currently integrated into clinical fitting software.

Lacking such a facility, users of currently available systems are provided with an analysis of the instantaneous integrity of the system. This occurs at two points: up to the speech processor, and up to a large part of the implanted electronics. First, alarm sounds, coloured lights or symbols on a display indicate sufficient battery power and integrity of the user programs stored in the speech processor. Second, some types of processor also signal whether telemetry indicates that the implant electronics are correctly communicating. This does not guarantee actual stimulation, but manufacturers claim that a responding implant is a positive test for the integrity of most of the implanted electronics. If communication is not established, users of some systems can place the transmitter over a receiver circuitry integrated in the processor housing or a separate device to check for RF output. If no RF output is present, the instruction manual guides the user through a series of corrective actions consisting of a systematic replacement of cables, microphone and transmitter coil. For this reason, it is advisable to provide each user with spare parts. However convenient and accurate, telemetry depends on functional implanted electronics. If telemetry fails because the implant does not respond, clinicians must consider further evaluating a non-stimulating implant with an independent procedure, such as recording surface potentials from the electrical stimulus artefact, as described in Chapter 3.

Aside from the issue of advanced detection of hardware problems, it needs to be said that up to now manufacturers have failed to provide implant centres with an objective means to test the quality of the microphone and (analogue) input stage of the processor. Obviously, microphones deteriorate gradually over time and so will performance, sometimes without the patient noticing. Even digital processors contain analogue input stages that may cause slight differences between processors that are audible to patients. At present, users, and parents of young users can marginally check the output of the microphone by watching a visual indication of the input circuit going into saturation as a function of input level and the sensitivity setting. Clinicians and parents can check the microphone by listening to it through earphones. What is needed is a comprehensive test similar to the standardized hearing instrument test procedure to check the frequency characteristic at several sound input levels, and objective figures of (harmonic) distortion. This need is increased for behind-the-ear speech processors that do not have an easily replaceable microphone.

Testing and optimizing the RF coupling

A strong coupling between transmitter and receiver coil is vital to avoid intermittency. However, as electronic parts become smaller and more energy efficient, the RF link will consume an increasingly larger part of the overall power requirement, so tuning it to maximum efficiency will extend battery life considerably. The RF power spent by the processor must be balanced against the supply voltage available in the implant, which cannot be less than a certain value depending on the particular stimulation strategy and sound input level to avoid the implant cutting out. Other factors affecting the required RF power are the current requirement of the subject, electrode impedance, skin thickness over the implant, the type of transmitter coil, the particular processor and even cable length (since each cable has a slightly different impedance). In some systems, clinicians can enter a diagnostic mode in which different configurations of components can be checked for optimal efficiency. Given a particular configuration, the processor can set the RF power to a minimum while continuously monitoring that the power is just sufficient to uphold the necessary supply voltage. An example is shown in Figure 2.1.

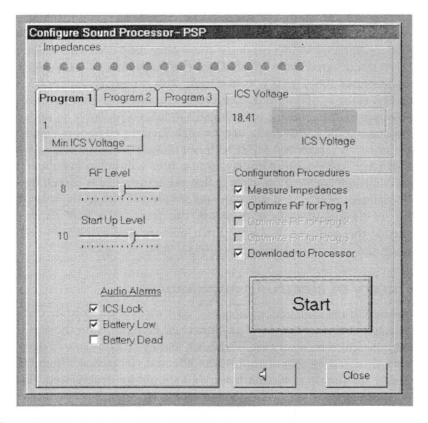

Figure 2.1. Optimization of the RF link in the CLARION fitting software. For each program, the implant supply voltage is monitored while changing the RF level used to start up the implant after being disconnected. The level is set so that the supply voltage is minimal yet acceptable. During use, the RF level is continuously minimized while monitoring supply voltage. Reprinted with permission from Advanced Bionics Corporation.

A general issue of RF signals is medical safety. The effects on the skin and other tissues in the head of the electromagnetic (EM) radiation generated by the transmitter coil is not covered by the technical manuals of the available systems, nor in any available study. Implant systems use carrier frequencies up to 50 MHz at energy levels that rule out hazardous ionization of molecules. However, non-ionizing side effects cannot be excluded. Unlike cell phones that pulse their RF output at a fixed, low frequency with possible effects on the organism, tissue heating is the only likely side effect in the case of cochlear implants. A thorough investigation of this issue is far beyond the scope of this chapter. Here only a rough estimate of the magnitude of the radiation will be made in comparison to that of cell phones, about which abundant literature exists. The CLARION system consumes more power than other systems to maintain sufficient power supply to its multiple current sources, so it creates a worst-case situation. Based on a measurement using a so-called top-detector which produces the voltage drop across a 50 ohm load for the rectified signal, we estimated that the transmitter of a CLARION 1.2 system generates about 0.16 W to the head. This is basically independent of stimulation strategy and stimulation levels. The estimate for a modern cell phone is approximately three times higher, and this is probably an underestimate because of the considerable antenna gain factor. Cell phones radiate at a higher frequency (about 900 MHz), so if cell phones create a marginal risk of tissue damage, the cochlear implant transmitter will do so even less. The argument against cochlear implants is that the transmitter is placed directly over a small area of skin, and that implants are used all day. In summary, local heating of tissues directly underneath the transmitter coil cannot be excluded at this moment. It is hoped that relevant data will be collected in the future and guidelines for manufacturers will be formulated.

Telemetry of electrode impedances

Lead wires and the connections between lead wires and electrode contacts are relatively frequent causes of malfunction, being outside the rigid and hermetically sealed receiver case. These can usually be adjusted to if detected properly, by avoiding stimulation of the affected electrodes. Open circuit electrodes are simply non-stimulating and should be deactivated. Widely spaced short-circuited electrodes create erratic electrical fields with potentially large effects on behavioural thresholds and the tonotopic order along the electrode array. These should also be deactivated. One may consider allowing stimulation on one of two short-circuited electrodes, if these are neighbouring, and the diagnosis is firm. Until recently, most systems only allowed electrode failures to be detected objectively by recording the surface potentials from the electrical artefact (Shallop, 1993; Mens et al., 1994a;

Shallop, 1997). The patient needed to be attached to a medically safe amplifier, and analysing the short circuits underlying a complex pattern of deviant surface potentials could be cumbersome.

The clinical fitting systems of all devices now feature a diagnostic telemetry mode in which malfunctioning electrodes can be detected in a short time and with minimal cooperation of the user. Basically, the voltage drop across the stimulating electrodes is measured at a particular point of the waveform, chosen to be representative of the overall amplitude, or at the end of the second phase where the output capacitor, if present, will be more or less discharged and of no effect. This momentary voltage divided by the current amplitude yields a measure of the impedance. It will depend on the integrity of the lead wires, properties of the electrode–tissue interface such as the effective surface (Ruddy and Loeb, 1995; Peeters et al., 1998) and tissue encapsulation, a possible air bubble covering the electrode, and the intervening anatomical structures that act as a volume conductor. Although complex in general, the resulting impedance is approximately resistive in the relevant frequency range (Spelman et al., 1982), thus allowing generalization of the measurement across the stimulus waveforms presented during normal use. To distinguish a genuine open circuit from biological causes of an increased impedance, a criterion needs to be set above which the electrode is flagged. This criterion will depend upon, amongst other things, the effective electrode surface. As an example, it is set at 20 kohm for the Nucleus 24 system with its relatively large electrodes, and 150 kohm in the case of the CLARION preformed array with small ball-shaped electrodes. Air bubbles often create a temporary open circuit intraoperatively which should not lead too easily to rejection of the device. If many electrodes are affected, it may be preferable to manipulate the electrode array slightly or even test it in saline after complete removal. It is not known if application of lubricants decreases the likelihood of dry electrodes.

In the default impedance test condition, each intracochlear electrode is tested separately in monopolar coupling against the extracochlear ground, and in this way open circuit electrodes will clearly stand out. Short-circuited electrodes, however, will only produce deviant (near zero) impedances if the affected non-stimulating electrode is connected to ground during the measurement. For this reason some devices feature not only a test in monopolar stimulation, but also one in 'common ground' in which all non-stimulating electrodes are connected to ground (Carter, 1997). Another option is to stimulate each electrode, one by one, in monopolar mode, and each time measure the voltage at all other non-stimulated electrodes. This results in a matrix of voltages, with the voltages of the active electrodes on the diagonal. Off-diagonal voltages are usually much less than half of diagonal voltages, as reactive polarization occurs in active electrodes only. Thus, only a short circuit will result in an off-diagonal voltage comparable to that on the diagonal. Using the pattern of voltages, the fitting software can automatically assign independent sets of short-circuited electrodes, if present.

Figure 2.2 shows the voltage table produced by the MED-EL CI.STUDIO+ software in graphical format. It illustrates a short circuit between electrodes 4 and 6. In the case of Figure 2.3, two sets of short-circuited electrodes are identified: A (electrodes 2, 3 and 5) and B (electrodes 9 and 11). In such a case the clinician has several options. If only a few short-circuited electrodes are distributed over the electrode array, all affected electrodes should be deactivated to avoid aberrant stimulation. If a block of (nearly) neighbouring electrodes is short-circuited, one option is to deactivate all electrodes of the block but the most apical, which has the effect of assigning one frequency band to the block of electrodes and stimulating all simultaneously. Usually, thresholds and comfort levels are lowest for the apical electrodes so one may hope that the most apical of the affected block dominates the percept.

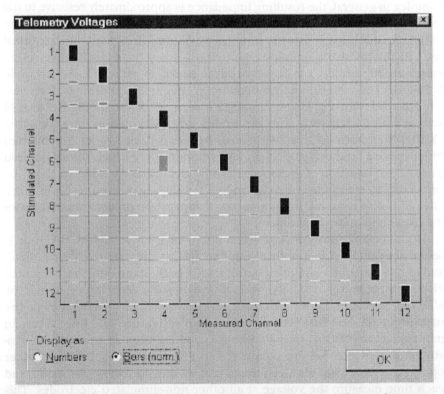

Figure 2.2. Voltage table produced by the MED-EL fitting software. This result suggests a short circuit between electrodes 4 and 6. The height of the bars is proportional to the voltage measured in the stimulated electrodes (on the diagonal) and the non-stimulated electrodes (off-diagonal). Reprinted with permission from MED-EL.

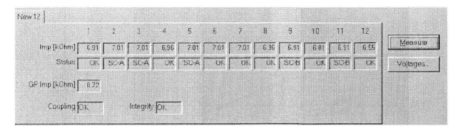

Figure 2.3. Impedance table produced by the MED-EL fitting software. Two sets of short-circuited electrodes are identified: A (electrodes 2, 3 and 5) and B (electrodes 9 and 11). Furthermore, an estimate of the ground path (GP) impedance is shown. Reprinted with permission from MED-EL.

Monopolar testing is only possible if the ground electrode is in good contact with tissue, otherwise all impedances will be high. If not all are high, an analysis of the impedances of a set of electrodes will show that the ground path is intact, and even enable an estimate of its impedance. In this way, changes in electrode impedances can be assigned locally near the intra-cochlear electrodes, or to a more diffuse process (Nopp et al., 2001).

For the purpose of establishing the integrity of the electrode array, it is not necessary to know the impedance with high accuracy. This may be different for research purposes, for instance when monitoring the effect of chemical deposits on the electrode surfaces over time. Several factors limit the accuracy of the impedance measurement. Typically, the stimulating current during impedance telemetry is at a low level, below threshold for most patients. One study (Nopp et al., 1998) suggests that this may lead to a slight underestimation of the impedance at higher amplitudes. The impedance of the stimulating electrodes measured *in vivo* was found to increase by about 20% each time the charge per phase was doubled. The authors assume capacitive and non-linear properties of the electrode interface and of the tissue. Further study is needed to verify this result in other systems. Accuracy is obviously affected by the quality of the analogue to digital converter (ADC) used for measuring the voltage, depending on the bit resolution and the way noise is cancelled. A more fundamental problem is that the current source inevitably is not ideal, which implies that the actual current level will deviate from the nominal current level set by the clinician, proportional to the load impedance. Figure 2.4 shows the ratio between actual and nominal current output that we found in our laboratory for a CLARION 1.2 research implant, at body temperature loaded with known resistors. If the impedance calculated by the fitting software is based on the nominal current level, it will be inaccurate, proportional to the deviations between actual and nominal current level. Even if currently available and future designs of the implanted current source will show smaller deviations on average, an on-chip calibration

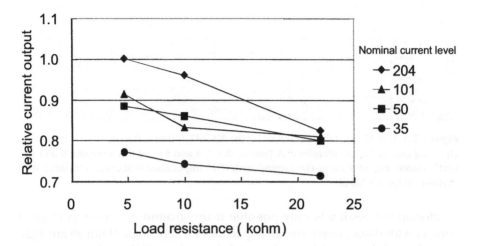

Figure 2.4. Ratio between the current delivered by a CLARION 1.2 implant and the nominal (command) current as a function of load resistance. Results are plotted for four different nominal current levels. No deviation was observed for a nominal current of 204 and a load of 5 kohm. Deviations up to 30% were found for smaller nominal current levels and higher loads. Measurements were made at 37°C.

of current source and ADC seems warranted, as individual implants that are out of specification cannot be excluded. Ideally, a high resolution ADC calibrated against a known voltage inside the implant would be used across a precision resistor in series with the patient load so as to establish the actual driving current and the voltage drop across the electrode in one and the same situation.

Compliance voltage telemetry

The data in Figure 2.4 imply that, even at low-to-intermediate current levels and load impedances, an actual current source may not output the required amplitude. In other words, it will often be slightly out of compliance. Any current source will be grossly out of compliance if the combination of required current and actual load exceeds the maximum supply voltage inside the implant. Some systems can detect when the implant has reached this compliance voltage while stimulating, other systems merely estimate the maximum current output on the basis of previously stored impedance values. In either case the clinician can take advantage of the information by knowing that setting the upper dynamic range above this point will not result in a further increase of loudness, but instead in an infinite compression of the upper part of the input sound level dynamic range. At present, compliance voltage is monitored during psychophysical testing on a channel by channel basis. Monitoring while processing live speech would seem to be required to detect instances when the implant is out of compliance during normal use. This is especially important if a simultaneous stimulation strategy is used, which drains supply voltage to a greater extent.

Although the term 'compliance voltage' may suggest a fixed voltage up to which current sources would be in compliance, in reality the output will level off gradually. We have demonstrated this for a CLARION 1.2 implant (Figure 2.5). This saturation will greatly affect the outcome of research that depends on the actual current output. But, even in fitting, the levelling of the loudness growth function may be a disadvantage. It is hoped that future designs of implanted current sources will correct this behaviour.

Assessing the distribution of the electrical field

A new form of telemetry is the assessment of the electrical field set up in the cochlea. This is accomplished by stimulating one channel and simultaneously measuring voltages on non-stimulated channels. This chapter will refer to these voltages as intracochlear electrode voltages (IEVs), in analogy to the surface potentials known as averaged electrode voltages (AEVs), both being the result of the electrical artefact. Previously it was mentioned that some systems already use IEVs to detect short circuits in the electrode array. In addition IEVs readily show the longitudinal voltage gradient along the

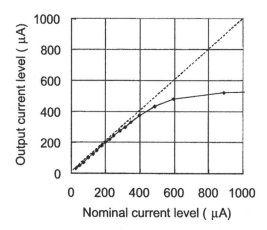

Figure 2.5. Output saturation of the CLARION 1.2 implant. As the nominal current level increases, the output current gradually deviates from the nominal value before the maximum (compliance) voltage of 7 V is reached. Measurements were made at 20°C with a 12 kohm load.

electrode array. This gradient may be related to how selectively each channel stimulates the nerve (Zierhofer et al., 1995; Mens et al., 1997). Previously, such measurements have been performed in animal and temporal bone studies using temporary probes (Ifukube and White, 1987; Jolly et al., 1996; Kral et al., 1998), the implanted electrode array itself (O'Leary et al., 1985), and intraoperatively using temporary probes (Kasper et al., 1991). Basically, these studies showed a voltage gradient that is about three times larger towards the base (with apical stimulation) than towards the apex (with basal stimulation). This suggests a preferential pathway through the basal openings. In a recent study (Kral et al., 1998), steeper gradients were found for quadrupolar stimulation (using out of phase currents on neighbouring channels), which also improved selectivity of stimulation as indicated by spatial tuning curves obtained from single units in the internal auditory meatus.

The membranous tissues and bony structures lining the scala tympani have a resistivity that is at least one order of magnitude larger than perilymph (Finley et al., 1991; Kasper et al., 1991). A considerable portion of the current injected at a certain point in the scala tympani will be shunted to the reference electrode (either intracochlear or extracochlear) without reaching the spiral ganglion and modiolus. The role of the scala tympani as a preferential pathway for current has been argued on the basis of the monotonic increase of AEVs with distance between active and reference electrode (Mens et al., 1994b) and of numerical models of volume conduction in the electrically stimulated ear (Mens et al., 1999; Briaire and Frijns, 2000). Thus, IEVs will predominantly pick up on these non-stimulating shunted currents. Nevertheless, IEVs may still be correlated to the width of excitation of a specific electrode for two reasons. First, if the width of excitation is in the order of the distance between stimulating and sensing electrodes, IEVs will also reflect currents that do stimulate the nerve after a certain amount of longitudinal spread. Second, it is reasonable to assume a (partial) trade-off between shunting and stimulating currents, which would imply that IEVs are always related to the width of the exciting field, however small. An obvious restriction on the usefulness of IEVs is that even with minimal current spread inside the scala tympani, selectivity can be virtually absent in some patients, for instance if the nerve is stimulated as a whole inside the modiolus (Frijns et al., 2000). In other words, a highly localized field as testified by IEVs is not a sufficient condition for good selectivity of stimulation.

We have measured IEVs intraoperatively to test the effect of the CLARION Electrode Positioning System™ (positioner) on the electrical field created by the HiFocus™ electrode array (Mens and Mulder, 2001). The positioner is used to bring each electrode contact closer to the modiolus, increasing the relative distance between the neural elements targeted by a specific electrode and the other electrodes. This is often referred to as a perimodiolar electrode array. A second benefit may result from the reduction of the volume of well-conducting perilymph around the electrode that increases the impedance of the longitudinal pathway in favour of radial currents towards the spiral ganglion. Third, the CLARION HiFocus electrode features protrusions at each side of the electrode surface which are said to act as 'di-electric partitions to reduce lateral current spread' (Lenarz et al., 1999). Intracochlear electrode voltages were collected intraoperatively using a research tool based on the CLARION Research Interface. All electrodes were referenced to the extracochlear ground. Figure 2.6 shows IEVs of one patient indicating a monotonous decrease of the electrical field strength both in apical and basal directions from the stimulated electrode, with some minor exceptions such as at electrode 5 in the apical direction. In this case, insertion of the positioner increased the (longitudinal) focusing of the field from almost all electrodes. However, we observed much smaller effects of the positioner in other patients. A conclusion to be considered is that the main advantage of

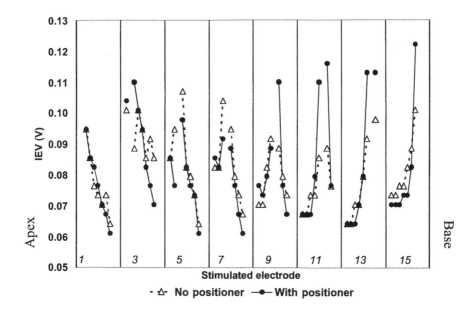

Figure 2.6. Intraoperative IEVs from a CLARION HiFocus array, before (triangles) and after (circles) insertion of the positioner. In the far left panel, electrode 1 (the most apical) is stimulated and IEVs are shown from electrodes 3–15. In the far right panel, electrode 15 (the most basal) is stimulated and IEVs are shown from electrodes 1–13. The electrode numbers are placed at about the location of the stimulated electrode in each panel and left to right is apical to basal in all panels. For convenience, only odd-numbered electrodes (for the 1.2 electrode array called 'medial' electrodes) were included. Measurements were made at 204 current units (about 160 µA).

the perimodiolar array investigated is the small distance between electrodes and neural elements, and that the effect on the focusing of the field is minor on average. The value of IEVs in measuring channel selectivity remains to be investigated. Intracochlear electrode voltages are more peripheral than, and therefore inferior to, direct neural indicators (Loeb et al., 1983; Kral et al., 1998), let alone psychophysical tests. However, they are easy to obtain and may provide additional information about the electrode array not contained in more central measures.

In one surgery out of the series mentioned above, grossly aberrant IEVs were found after insertion of the positioner, as shown in Figure 2.7. Voltages increased with distance between stimulated and recording electrode for some electrodes (for example stimulated electrode 1), which was not the case before insertion of the positioner. In addition, stapedial reflex thresholds were higher with the positioner. After reinsertion of the positioner, a more acceptable pattern of IEVs was found, and reflex thresholds were at about the level they were without the positioner. Postoperative X-rays showed normal position of the electrode array in both patients presented in Figures 2.6 and 2.7. With the increase of intricate surgical manoeuvres of the electrode array, IEVs may well become an integral part of the intraoperative

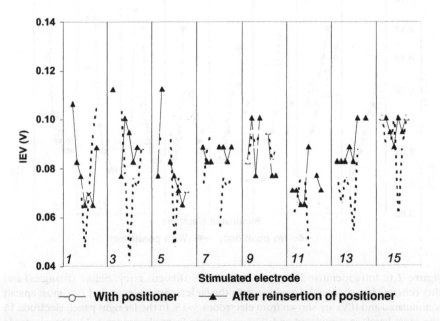

Figure 2.7. Aberrant intraoperative IEVs from a CLARION HiFocus electrode array. The positioner was inserted (circles), removed and inserted a second time (triangles). Measurements were made at 101 current units (about 80 µA).

test battery, whether to quantify current spread, or merely to check for abnormal electrical fields created by a deviant placement of the electrode array. In this sense, IEVs can conveniently replace AEVs, which have been shown in some cases to signal unusual electrode configurations or cochlear malformations or both.

A look into the future

Telemetry circuits have already increased the quality of modern cochlear implant systems in several ways. They have removed part of the uncertainty about the technical integrity of both external and internal components, during surgery, during clinical troubleshooting as well as during everyday use. Telemetry has begun already to contribute to the fitting of young children by providing preliminary data on the responsiveness of the peripheral auditory system. Currently available systems obviously differ in the type of telemetry-based features, and not all features are equally necessary. Most vital is the possibility of evaluating the technical integrity of the implanted receiver during surgery and during postoperative fitting sessions. All systems offer this. What is not consistently offered to the clinician is the possibility of ruling out more trivial but frequent causes of an absent response of the implanted electronics. These include a broken cable, defective transmitter coil or a weak coupling to the implant. Ideally, these different modes of failure would be logged in the processor and accessed by the user and by the clinician in a direct consultation or through a remote (telephone) connection. Although telemetry may become quite advanced at detecting failures, it seems important for a clinical centre to collect surface potentials routinely, as these are device independent and may show intermittent failures and deviant stimulation patterns missed by telemetry.

Telemetry of electrode impedances is another vital feature already present in all systems. It is desirable to be able to test electrodes not only in monopolar, but also in bipolar modes of stimulation to diagnose complex short circuits. As far as impedances affect the behaviour of current sources during psychophysical testing, on-board calibration is called for. Specification of the output in terms of charge per phase instead of device-specific current units is another desirable feature. This would facilitate direct comparison of different research studies.

Some fitting systems provide a warning to the clinician that the implant is not able to supply the requested output during threshold and comfort level testing. To avoid a limited dynamic range because of this compliance limitation, the clinician may take corrective action, for instance by increasing the pulse width. However convenient, it is likely that a test on a channel by channel basis underestimates the compliance problems that may arise in the case of simultaneous stimulation. Ideally, the system would monitor for compliance problems continuously during the delivery of complex signals at a loud level.

As objective measures become increasingly important in fitting young children, telemetry will be expected to provide a convenient access to neural responses. The intracochlear registration of the compound action potential will possibly be complemented with that of potentials from the brainstem and the auditory cortex, either transient or steady state. One can envisage extra electrodes being placed for this purpose. These would be very long unipolar electrodes attached to the receiver/stimulator, similar to the separate ground electrode already used in some systems, but placed further away.

In the future, telemetry will tighten the loop between fitting and performance even further, increasing the quality of cochlear implants in individual patients as well as over generations of increasingly refined systems.

Acknowledgements

Representatives of the manufacturers mentioned in this chapter have kindly provided additional information. Specifically Patrick Boyle and Dzemal Gazibegovic (Advanced Bionics Corporation), Peter Nopp (MED-EL) and Barry Nevison (Cochlear Limited) are gratefully acknowledged for scrutinizing the facts in Table 2.1. Remaining errors are the responsibility of the author. Harry van der Zwart of our technical department was instrumental in assessing the RF issue.

References

Briaire JJ, Frijns JH (2000) Field patterns in a 3D tapered spiral model of the electrically stimulated cochlea. Hear Res 148: 18–30.

Carter P (1997) Determining electrode faults using different stimulation modes. Presented at XVI World Congress of ORL – Head and Neck Surgery, Sydney, Australia.

Finley CC, Wilson BS, White MW (1991) Models of neural responsiveness to electrical stimulation. In Miller J, Spelman F (eds) Cochlear Implants: Models of the Electrically Stimulated Ear. New York: Springer Verlag, pp. 55–93.

Frijns JH, Briaire JJ, Schoonhoven R (2000) Integrated use of volume conduction and neural models to simulate the response to cochlear implants. Simulation Practice and Theory 8: 75–97.

Ifukube T, White RL (1987) Current distributions produced inside and outside the cochlea from a scala tympani electrode array. IEEE Trans Biomed Eng 34: 883–90.

Jolly CN, Spelman FA, Clopton BM (1996) Quadrupolar stimulation for cochlear prostheses: modeling and experimental data. IEEE Trans Biomed Eng 43: 857–65.

Kasper A, Pelizzone M, Montandon P (1991) Intracochlear potential distribution with intracochlear and extracochlear electrical stimulation in humans. Ann Otol Rhinol Laryngol 100: 812–16.

Kral A, Hartmann R, Mortazavi D, Klinke R (1998) Spatial resolution of cochlear implants: the electrical field and excitation of auditory afferents. Hear Res 121: 11–28.

Lenarz T, Kuzma J, Maltan AA (1999) The HiFocus© electrode system. Presented at Conference on Implantable Auditory Prostheses, Pacific Grove CA, USA.

Loeb GE, White MW, Jenkins WM (1983) Biophysical considerations in electrical stimulation of the auditory nervous system. Ann N Y Acad Sci 405: 123–36.

Mens LHM, Oostendorp TF, Van den Broek P (1994a) Identifying electrode failures with cochlear implant generated surface potentials. Ear Hear 15: 330–8.

Mens LHM, Oostendorp TF, Van den Broek P (1994b) Cochlear implant generated surface potentials: current spread and side effects. Ear Hear 15: 339–45.

Mens LHM, Van den Broek P (1997) Telemetry of longitudinal current spread: does it show spatial selectivity? Presented at Conference on Implantable Auditory Prostheses, Pacific Grove CA, USA.

Mens LHM, Huiskamp G, Van den Broek P, Oostendorp TF (1999) Modeling surface potentials from intra-cochlear electrical stimulation. Scand Audiol 28: 249–55.

Mens LHM, Mulder JJS (2001) Telemetry of intracochlear electrode voltages (IEVs) in users of the CLARION system. Presented at 2nd International Symposium and Workshop on Objective Measures in Cochlear Implantation, Lyon, France.

Nopp P, Kerber M, Zierhofer C, Brill S (1998) Impedance telemetry as a means of implant evaluation. Presented at First International Symposium and Workshop on Objective Measures in Cochlear Implantation, Nottingham, UK.

Nopp P, Jaeger A, Meinschad P (2001) Advanced impedance telemetry using MED-EL's CI.STUDIO+ software. Presented at 2nd International Symposium and Workshop on Objective Measures in Cochlear Implantation, Lyon, France.

O'Leary SJ, Black RC, Clark GM (1985) Current distributions in the cat cochlea: a modeling and electrophysiological study. Hear Res 18: 273–81.

Peeters S, Van Immerseel L, Zarowski A, Houben V, Govaerts P, Offeciers E (1998) New developments in cochlear implants. Acta Otorhinolaryngol Belg 52: 115–27.

Ruddy HA, Loeb GE (1995) Influence of materials and geometry on fields produced by cochlear electrode arrays. Med Biol Eng Comput 33: 793–801.

Shallop JK (1993) Objective electrophysiological measures from cochlear implant patients. Ear Hear 14: 58–63.

Shallop JK (1997) Objective measurements and the audiological management of cochlear implant patients. Adv Otorhinolaryngol 53: 85–111.

Spelman FA, Clopton BM, Pfingst BE (1982) Tissue impedance and current flow in the implanted ear. Implications for the cochlear prosthesis. Ann Otol Rhinol Laryngol 98(Suppl), pp. 3–8.

Zierhofer CM, Hochmair-Desoyer IJ, Hochmair ES (1995) Electronic design of a cochlear implant for multichannel high-rate pulsatile stimulation strategies. IEEE Trans on Rehab Engineering 3: 112–16.

CHAPTER 3

Averaged electrode voltage measurements in patients with cochlear implants

JON K SHALLOP, PAUL CARTER, GAIL FEINMAN, BRUCE TABOR

Contents

- Introduction.
- Definition of averaged electrode voltages.
- AEV methodology.
- AEV results.
- The Crystal Integrity Test System.
- Discussion.
- Conclusions.

Introduction

There are various ways to evaluate the integrity of the internal components of a multichannel cochlear implant. Adults and older children can typically provide adequate behavioural responses and descriptions, which enable the subjective verification of device function. However, occasionally the need arises to differentiate among behavioural, physiological and device-related problems. We first described some basic measurement aspects of averaged electrode voltages (AEVs) in two previous publications (Heller et al., 1991 and 1993). Since then the measurement of far-field surface voltages resulting from the stimulation currents of a cochlear implant has been used by several authors as a method to assess the integrity of the components of cochlear implants (Almqvist et al., 1993; Mens et al., 1993, 1994a and 1994b; Shallop, 1993a and 1993b; Shallop et al., 1993; Shipp et al., 1993; Mahoney and Rotz Proctor, 1994; Peterson et al., 1995).

Averaged electrical voltages provide an indirect measure of stimulator and electrode function; therefore the stimulation and recording techniques as well as the distribution of current in the cochlea influence the results. We have investigated the effects of recording amplifier parameters, electrode placement and stimulus parameters on AEVs. In this chapter, we will describe the results from our investigations and detail a recommended technique in order to minimize the distortion of AEVs.

Definition of averaged electrode voltages

When a cochlear implant is activated, the current between specific electrodes produces a measurable voltage (electrode voltage or EV) which can be measured in real time as a far-field potential. However, the EV amplitude may not be sufficiently above background noise levels to enable accurate measurements. Averaged electrode voltages (AEVs) are EVs averaged over time. They can be recorded far-field – on the surface of the head. However, AEVs are influenced by various factors, which we have grouped into the categories: stimulation parameters, acquisition parameters and anatomical and/or physiological considerations. These factors are detailed further in Table 3.1.

A simple way to record the far-field electrode voltages from a cochlear implant is with selective amplification through an isolation amplifier and display on an oscilloscope. This method has been used to verify the integrity or malfunction of the internal components of single and multichannel cochlear implants. However, this method is limited by signal to noise considerations and

Table 3.1. Summary of factors which have a significant effect on surface recorded AEVs in cochlear implant users

Stimulation Parameters
    Current level
    Mode of stimulation: monopolar, bipolar and common ground
    Pulse width

Acquisition Parameters
    Amplifier gain
    Amplifier bandwidth
    Averager sampling rate
    Averager triggering
    Recording electrode montage
    Radio frequency interference

Anatomical and Physiological Considerations
    Electrode array placement
    Cochlear anatomy (normal vs abnormal)
    Temporal bone conductivity (e.g. affected by meningitis, otosclerosis)

the cooperation of the patient. Background EEG and EMG make it difficult to observe real time EVs accurately below about 10 µV peak to peak, due to amplifier noise, patient activity (EMG) level and radio frequency (RF) interference. We have employed signal averaging to improve the signal to noise ratio to obtain more accurate measurements. In this chapter we will describe different methods for obtaining AEVs and emphasize the importance of using stimulation and acquisition parameters that optimize these measurements and minimize distortion. We will first describe our experience with AEV measurements from the Nucleus® CI22M device. These techniques have applications to other cochlear implant devices including CLARION®, MED-EL, Laura and MXM. We will end the chapter with a description of the Crystal Integrity Test System, which uses many of the techniques we describe in the early parts of the chapter.

AEV methodology

Normative data for Nucleus CI22M

The population we describe consists of postlingually deafened adults (>18 years old) who received the Nucleus 22 channel (standard or Mini) cochlear implant. It was verified that each subject had all active electrodes intra-cochlear based on the subject's behavioural responses to stimulation on all electrodes, the operative record of the surgeon and in some cases by post-operative radiographic studies. Additionally, any patients with known cochlear anomalies and/or retrocochlear pathology were excluded from this normative group. The average time of implant use was 25 months (range = 6-61) and the average subject age was 52 years (range = 25-82). The normative group included 14 females and 16 males. Average insertion depth of the electrode array was 23 mm (full insertion of the 22 active electrodes and 10 stiffening rings is 25 mm) with a standard deviation of 2 mm, based on the operative reports for each subject. The ear of implantation was left in 14 cases, and right in 16.

Stimulation equipment and parameters

The stimulation equipment set-up is illustrated in Figure 3.1. The cochlear implant is activated using the standard computer interface system for the Nucleus 22 channel cochlear implant device. An IBM compatible personal computer with a Cochlear Ltd interface card (IF4) is connected to a dual processor interface (DPI) and a speech processor (Mini Speech Processor (MSP) or Spectra 22). The output of the speech processor is connected to the patient's headset (HS6) or a test headset (HS7). A triggering cable needs to be connected from the audio output jack of the DPI to the external input of the

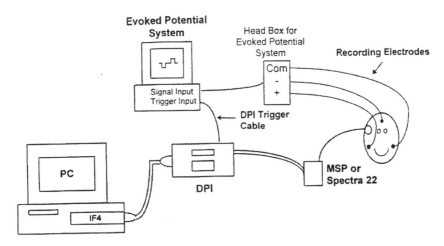

Figure 3.1. Equipment diagram for CI22M AEV recordings with Nicolet C4. Stimulation of the cochlear implant is controlled by the proprietary software (DPS 6.0x or WIN-DPS R116) on an IBM compatible computer. An interface card is required.

evoked potential system. Because the DPI audio output is a transistor transistor logic (TTL)[1] signal that is synchronized to the stimuli, it provides an efficient trigger signal for the evoked potential system. Stimulation was controlled using a version of the Cochlear Ltd Diagnostic Programming Software (DPS version 6.125) which allows for stimulation in various bipolar modes (BP, BP+1, ... to BP+20) and common ground mode (CG) (Crosby et al., 1984). Appendix 1.1 to Chapter 1 shows diagrams of different stimulation modes. The pulse width is typically 200 µs/phase and current level can be varied, but should never exceed the patient's maximum comfort level. We typically use a stimulation pulse rate of 250 Hz. The stimulation burst duration is 1,000 ms and the interburst duration is 1 ms, resulting in a nearly continuous pulse train at 250 Hz. The output from the implant is a negative-leading, charge-balanced biphasic waveform.

Acquisition equipment and parameters

The evoked potential system was triggered externally by the control signal from the implant programming system using a trigger cable as described above. Analysis parameters for the evoked potential system (Nicolet Compact Four) typically included: preamplifier sensitivity of 10 µV, bandpass filtering

---

[1] TTL (Transistor Transistor Logic) is an engineering term which specifies a triggering pulse voltage of ± 5V from one device (for example, cochlear implant interface) used to synchronize another device (for example, oscilloscope or signal averager).

of 1 to 10,000 Hz, analysis time of 10 ms, artefact reject off, and the averager trigger was set to external. The number of averages necessary is dependent on the state of the subject and the overall amplitude of the AEVs for that subject. When subjects are 'quiet' and the AEVs are large, 25 averages are usually adequate, which takes about 1 s per electrode. However, when the subject is awake and movement artefacts are likely, or when AEV amplitudes are small, we typically average 200 samples (about 6 s per electrode). Each electrode is usually tested in sequence from base (electrode 1) to apex (electrode 22) after making sure that all signals to be used never exceed maximum comfort levels.

During AEV measurements, the evoked potential system amplifies and filters the signals (including a low-pass RF filter) picked up by the recording electrodes on the scalp. These amplified analogue signals are then converted into digital signals and averaged across multiple samples. The averager analysis time and the number of samples (512) per time window determine the sampling rate for each AEV acquisition. Thus the combination of a 10 ms analysis time and 512 sampling points results in a sampling rate of 51,200 Hz which is sufficient for the preamplifier bandwidth of 1–10,000 Hz. This sampling rate adequately resolves the typical stimulation pulse width that we recommend of 200 μs per phase at a rate of 250 Hz. A minimum of 10 sampling points per phase is obtained under these conditions. For all of our normative measurements, we adhere to the fundamental principle of the Nyqvist theorem, which specifies that for an accurate reconstruction of an analogue signal, the digital sampling rate must be at least twice the highest frequency contained in the signal.

For some of the test measurements, we have obtained AEVs from a Nucleus 22 channel implant suspended in a phosphate buffered saline test tank. The electrode array was coiled around a small glass rod to simulate curvature within the cochlea. Voltage waveforms were recorded directly from the output terminals of the implant and from electrodes in the saline tank on opposite sides of the electrode array. These configurations were intended to simulate the montages used in the surface recordings from the adult subjects with implants.

Recording electrode montages

Figure 3.2 illustrates the three recording electrode montages that we have used in our investigations for the adult cochlear implant subjects. For each montage, the ipsilateral mastoid (with reference to the cochlear implant ear) was used as the positive non-inverting input to the preamplifier. The vertex (Cz) was used as the negative inverting input for montage A and the ground electrode was placed on the forehead at FPz. For montage B we used FPz as

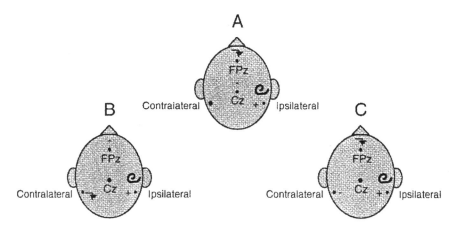

Figure 3.2. Recording electrode montages.

the negative input and the contralateral mastoid served as the ground. For montage C we used the contralateral mastoid as the negative input and the ground was FPz. The recording electrode locations were cleansed with isopropyl alcohol and lightly abraded with Omni Prep™. Surface silver/silver chloride disk electrodes with electrode paste (MediTrace EEG SOL™) were taped in place with plastic adhesive tape. Recording electrode impedances were verified to be less than 2,000 ohms. The surface recording electrodes were the input to the evoked potential system.

AEV results

AEV amplitudes and current level

The amplitude of the cochlear implant stimulation will obviously affect the amplitude of the measured AEVs. In Figure 3.3, we demonstrate this effect with a test implant in a saline test tank. The electrode array was suspended in 2% buffered saline solution and the implant was activated as described above in a bipolar stimulation mode. The biphasic output programming current level of the device ranged from 30 to 239 (approximately equivalent to 40–1,500 µA peak). The active recording electrodes were placed 2 cm on either side of electrode 1 of the cochlear implant electrode array. The measured AEVs ranged from 40 to 2,500 µV peak-to-peak over the range of output currents. This result illustrates that the Nucleus cochlear implant current level scale is non-linear and actual current in µA is related to programming current level by the expression:

Current (mA) $\approx 0.02 \times 1.01858^{CL}$

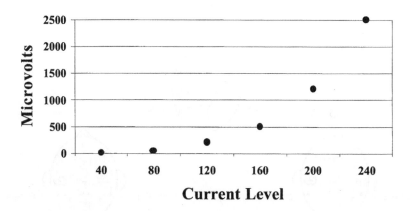

Figure 3.3. Amplitude growth of AEVs at various current levels of a test CI22M cochlear implant. The implant was placed in a saline filled test tank; see text for additional details. The amplitude growth is non-linear. These amplitudes were measured for bipolar stimulation, which consistently produced biphasic waveforms with equal amplitudes of each phase across the current range.

In the formula, CL represents the current level in programming units used in the Cochlear Ltd DPS software. The actual current output for each cochlear implant varies slightly and a calibration table can be obtained from Cochlear Ltd for any specific device. In order to minimize the impact of background noise from adult subjects, we select current levels that will produce AEVs of sufficient peak-to-peak amplitude that exceed the background noise, but we never exceed the maximum comfort level of awake cochlear implant patients.

Effects of stimulation mode

Typical findings in BP+1 mode

Figure 3.4 shows the AEV responses for the 20 active electrodes of an adult patient (LH) in stimulation mode BP+1 at a current level of approximately 300 µA peak (programming CL of 126). Most of our testing in bipolar modes was done with this current level because it represents about 20% of the CI22M device output range and this level is typically audible but not too loud for many cochlear implant users. This patient had an unremarkable cochlear implant surgery, and all 22 active electrodes plus the 10 stiffening rings (32/32) of the array were judged to be intracochlear by the surgeon. The AEVs show a negative-leading (non-inverted) series of waveforms, which decrease in amplitude from base to apex. Also note that there were no phase reversals in the complete set of responses for this subject. This pattern was

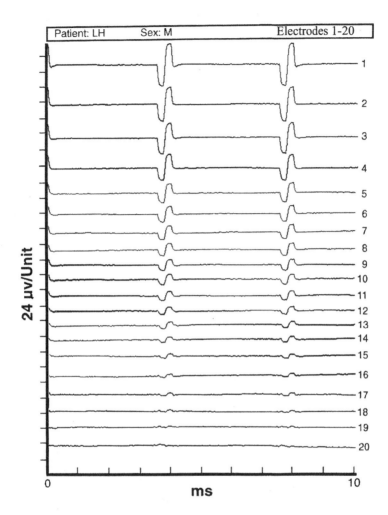

Figure 3.4. BP+1 AEV responses from adult cochlear implant patient LH for electrodes 1 to 20. Stimulation was at a programming current level of 126. Note how the AEV amplitudes decrease as the stimulated electrode advances from base to apex of the cochlea.

observed in many (14/30) of the normative patients we have studied in BP+1. The AEV amplitude decreases monotonically as the electrode stimulation site moves toward the apex of the cochlea. In Figure 3.5 we illustrate the amplitudes (μV peak to peak) as measured for each of the electrodes (1 to 20) in BP+1 mode for subject LH. The programming stimulation current was 126 for each electrode. The AEV amplitudes for LH are typical of the average AEV amplitudes shown in Figure 3.6 as reported for 30 adults by Shallop (1993a). These results are similar to those reported by Shipp (1993) for 25 adults.

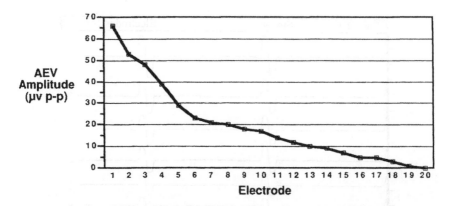

Figure 3.5. AEV amplitudes from Figure 3.4 plotted across the electrode array. The peak-to-peak amplitude decreases from about 65 µV for electrode 1 to less than 5 µV on electrode 20.

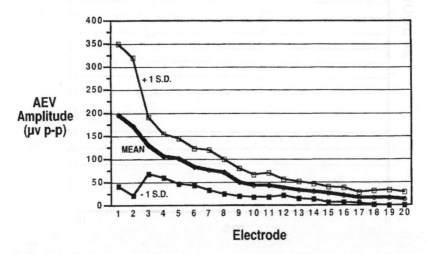

Figure 3.6. Mean BP+1 AEV amplitude normative data for the 30 adults reported in Shallop (1993b). The mean peak-to-peak amplitude decreases from about 200 µV for electrode 1 to about 5 µV on electrode 20.

There is good agreement between these two studies reporting adult results, in comparison to the larger AEV amplitudes reported for children by Mahoney and Rotz Proctor (1994).

Atypical findings in BP+1 mode

There are three AEV patterns that have typically been observed in bipolar and monopolar stimulation modes. These are illustrated schematically in Figure 3.7. The stimulus is a charge balanced negative-leading biphasic current

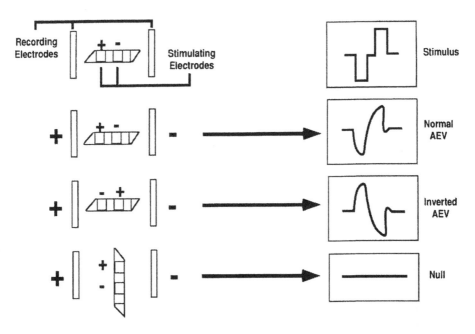

Figure 3.7. Three AEV patterns shown for a charge-balanced stimulus. Reversing the current flow will cause the far-field recorded AEVs to invert. A null response can occur if the current flow is parallel to the plane of the recording electrodes.

pulse stimulating adjacent electrodes (BP mode is illustrated in this case). The normal AEV occurs as illustrated when the polarity sequence is as shown in relation to the recording electrodes. However, if for some reason the stimulation electrodes are reversed or the current path is reversed, the resultant recorded AEV will be inverted as shown. Moreover, if the stimulation electrodes (or current flow) are in a parallel plane relative to the recording electrodes, then a null in the AEV will be observed.

In some of the normative subjects (5/30), there were one or more phase reversals in the AEV sequence from base to apex. This finding is illustrated for patient DW in Figure 3.8. This patient had a known history of otosclerosis as the aetiology of his hearing loss, as well as a traumatic head injury. Note that the waveforms are non-inverted and negative-leading on the basal electrodes 1 to 8. An apparent null response and a phase reversal occurs at electrode 9 and then the AEVs are positive-leading (inverted) until electrode 17 where there is another apparent null response. Such null responses are often seen on apical electrodes in narrow bipolar modes. They apparently result from geometric changes in the orientation of the voltage dipole. At electrode 17 there is another phase reversal, and the AEVs are then negative-leading. The amplitude and phase of AEVs obtained from DW in BP+1 are summarized in

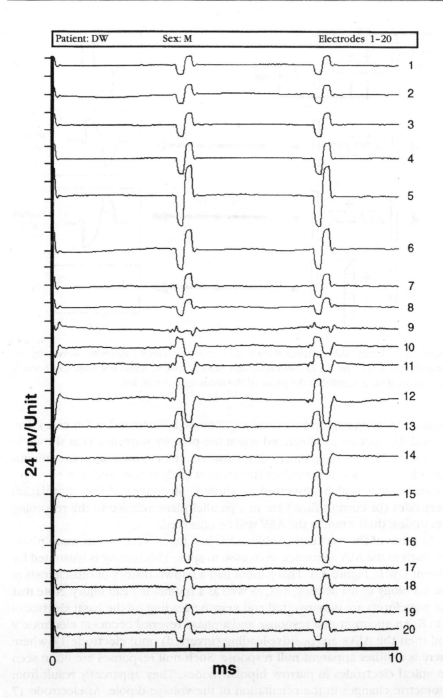

Figure 3.8. Unusual pattern of AEVs for patient DW. This illustrates a distinct null response at electrodes 9 and 17, and phase reversals.

Figure 3.9. These results demonstrate how erratic AEV amplitude patterns can be when obtained in BP+1 mode. Note that the phase reversed AEVs (positive-leading) are plotted as negative amplitudes in order to clearly illustrate the phase reversals.

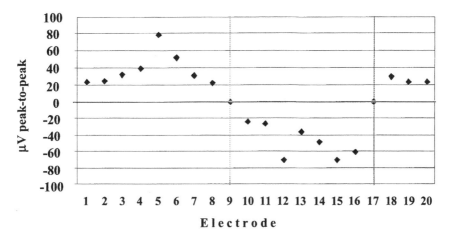

Figure 3.9. AEV amplitudes and phases from Figure 3.8 plotted across the electrode array. The phase reversal pattern is unique for this patient, who has a history of otosclerosis and head trauma. AEV positive values (µV peak-to-peak) are plotted for waveforms with a negative-leading voltage, and the negative AEV values are plotted for waveforms with a positive-leading waveform. Note the null points at electrodes 9 and 17.

Effects of common ground mode

Some clinicians have preferred to program younger CI22M cochlear implant patients in common ground mode. However, we will stress the need to be aware of how this mode can distort AEVs. We have found that common ground mode with any cochlear implant device can cause significant amounts of distortion of AEVs in comparison to bipolar modes.

In a 'tank test' experiment to compare modes, we used the electrode array of the Nucleus 22 channel mini receiver/stimulator. The array was wrapped around a short glass rod (diameter = 3 mm) in order to approximate the coiled shape of the cochlea. This array was placed in a small saline tank (10 × 10 × 10 cm) and driven by the receiver/stimulator at a current level of 200 and a pulse width of 200 µs/phase. The rate was 250 Hz. Various active electrodes were stimulated using the modes common ground, BP+1 and BP+5. Prior to measuring the AEVs, the current output of the implant was measured directly to confirm that the biphasic pulses were always charge balanced in all of the stimulation modes. Averaged electrode voltages were then measured in various stimulation modes with one of the recording electrodes approximately 3 cm from the electrode array and the second approximately 7 cm on the opposite side of the spiralled electrode array. AEVs were always symmetric balanced biphasic pulses in the various bipolar modes. However, common ground would frequently produce asymmetric waveforms, especially near a null point, as shown in Figure 3.10 for the sequential set of active electrodes 13, 14, 15 and 16. This sequence was selected because of the null observed in common ground, which was not present for these same electrodes in any bipolar mode. As the centre tracing in Figure 3.10 demonstrates, the output to all four electrodes was charge balanced, but the far-field AEVs were distorted in common ground mode and not in the bipolar modes. Figure 3.11 compares the AEVs measured in the tank test set-up for common ground (CG) versus bipolar (BP) modes of stimulation at two pulse widths (100 μs/phase and 400 μs/phase). Note that the bipolar stimulation AEV is symmetrical but that the two CG AEVs appear to be monophasic. Again, this is an artefact of using CG stimulation mode to record AEVs, which we do not recommend.

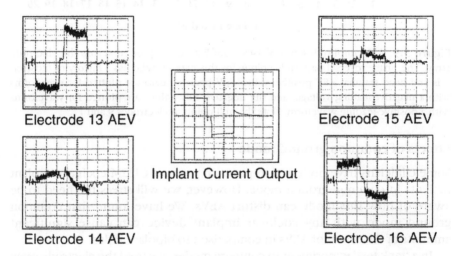

Figure 3.10. AEVs recorded using CG mode for a test CI22M in saline. This illustrates clear null points on electrodes 14 and 15. The stimulation current was a charge balanced biphasic pulse at a current level of 200 with a pulse width of 200 μs/phase for all recordings. In various bipolar modes, we never observed null points. However, as shown in this figure, AEVs in common ground mode will typically give voltage null points which may result in the incorrect interpretation of electrode function.

In the second part of our studies, we measured AEVs in common ground and a bipolar stimulation mode (using electrode 1 as the indifferent) in 19 of our 30 normative subjects. The AEVs were measured for pulse widths of 400, 200, 100 and 50 μs/phase at a stimulation rate of 250 Hz. The analysis time

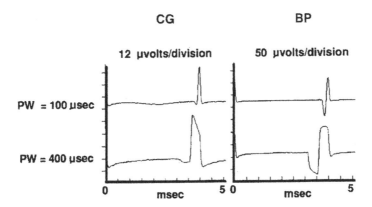

Figure 3.11. Comparison of AEVs recorded using CG and BP modes for a test CI22M in saline. This illustrates how it is possible to observe 'monophasic' AEVs in CG when the BP AEVs are normal. The stimulation current was a charge balanced biphasic pulse at a current level of 228 with pulse widths of 100 and 400 µs/phase. The sampling rate adequately resolves the waveforms. This again illustrates that AEVs in common ground mode will result in artefactual abnormal AEVs.

was 5 ms and AEVs were measured on electrodes 20 and 5. In order to compare the results across subjects, the amplitude of each AEV phase was normalized with respect to the peak-to-peak amplitude, and then the difference between the normalized amplitude of each phase was calculated. The means and standard deviations for each condition are shown in Figure 3.12. These results clearly demonstrate the distortion of AEVs that are measured in common ground. The phase 1 versus phase 2 mean amplitude differences ranged from 23% to 34% in common ground, in contrast to the same measures in bipolar where phase 1 and phase 2 were nearly identical (2.5%–10% difference). The mean 10% difference at the pulse width of 50 µs/phase demonstrates a trend that we have observed when the signal averager sampling rate cannot adequately resolve the stimulation pulse width.

An example of distorted AEVs in common ground versus BP+1 is shown in Figure 3.13. These AEVs were obtained from an adult cochlear implant patient (CN) who had a full insertion of all active electrodes and all ten of the array stiffening rings. We used the same active electrode (8) in the bipolar + 1 and common ground modes at the same current level (65 µA peak) and pulse width of 400 µs/phase. The common ground (upper tracing) AEV is distorted, with the first phase being larger in amplitude than the second distorted phase. The AEV in BP+1 is symmetrical and undistorted. This example is illustrative of the waveform morphologies measured for the subjects in this experiment, and another example of why common ground mode AEVs should only be used with the understanding that the waveforms will be distorted.

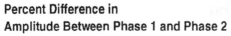

Percent Difference in
Amplitude Between Phase 1 and Phase 2

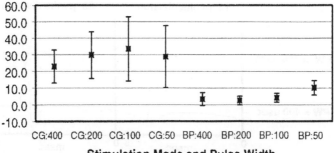

Stimulation Mode and Pulse Width

Figure 3.12. Percentage of AEV phase 1 versus phase 2 amplitude differences observed for CG and BP modes. Pulse widths were 400, 200, 100 and 50 µs/phase. The CG mode clearly produced more distortion in these 19 adult subjects with a CI22M cochlear implant.

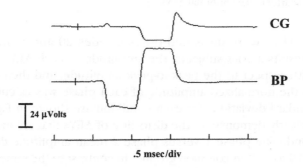

Figure 3.13. AEVs in BP+1 and CG for adult subject CN. These AEVs were obtained on electrode 8, which functioned normally in her speech processor programs. The CG tracing shows phase and amplitude distortion while the BP+1 AEV is normal.

Effects of wide bipolar modes

The advantages of wide bipolar and monopolar modes for the measurement of AEVs have been described (Heller et al., 1993). Their findings from a few subjects demonstrate that the amplitude of the AEVs increase as the stimulation mode increases from BP to BP+20 (effectively monopolar) and as the site of stimulation moves from apex to base. In Figure 3.14, the AEVs of adult subject SG are shown for samples obtained using his basal active electrode (electrode 1) as the indifferent electrode for all of the remaining electrodes (2 to 22) of the electrode array. The remaining stimulation parameters were identical to the BP+1 parameters described above except that the current level was reduced to 65 µA (programming current level of 50) in order to

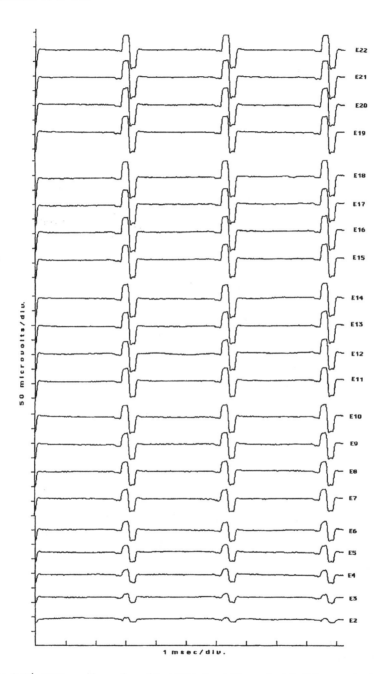

Figure 3.14. AEV waveforms for subject SG in 'variable modes'. In this case electrode 1 is used as the indifferent electrode and all other active stimulation electrodes are paired to electrode 1, in sequence from electrodes 2 to 22. The current level used was 50 and the pulse width was 200 μs/phase. Note how the amplitudes of the AEVs gradually increase from base to apex as the stimulation mode widens, even though the current level is fixed.

avoid uncomfortable sensations in wide stimulation modes. These AEVs were also obtained using the stimulogram technique (Figure 3.15) developed by Almqvist et al. (1993). Note, in Figures 3.14 and 3.15, that as the bipolar modes widen from base to apex, the AEV amplitudes increase in proportion to the mode width until about electrode 16 when the AEVs plateau at about 75 μV. The normative data obtained from our 30 adult subjects using this technique are shown in Figure 3.16. The AEV amplitude values for SG are shown for reference, and the thicker line represents the mean AEV values. The ±1 standard deviation (SD) values are displayed as the dotted lines. The mean AEV values increase from basal to apical electrodes, reaching maximal between electrodes 14 and 16 at 130–140 μV. These amplitudes of the AEVs in widening bipolar modes with the current fixed at 65 μA were considerably larger than those we have measured in BP+1 at a current level of 300 μA (see Figure 3.6).

Effects of amplifier gain

It is important to use the proper level of preamplifier gain when assessing AEVs. With our equipment, we typically set the preamplifier gain at a sensitivity of 1,000 μV, which corresponds to a gain of 120,000. This gain is usually sufficient to measure AEVs above 100 μV and below 1,000 μV. When AEVs exceed 1,000 μV, the amplifier sensitivity must be reduced to avoid peak clipping. When AEVs are less than 100 μV, the amplifier sensitivity needs to be increased to improve the resolution of the waveforms; AEV amplitudes that we have measured typically range from 10 to 700 μV peak to peak.

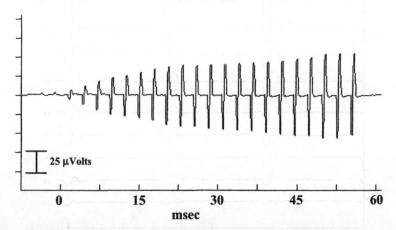

Figure 3.15. AEV waveforms for subject SG plotted as a stimulogram. In this series, the stimulation was a rapid series like a 'burst' of sequential pulses quickly stimulating electrodes 2 to 22 with electrode 1 as the indifferent electrode. This is the methodology used by Almqvist et al., 1993. The AEVs are recorded in a single time window of 60 ms that averages the electrode voltages in about 1 second.

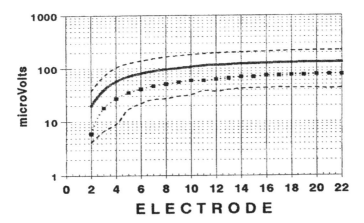

Figure 3.16. Mean 'variable mode' AEV amplitude normative data for 30 adults. Electrode 1 was used as the indifferent electrode. Current level was 50. The mean amplitude of the responses is shown as the thick solid line with ± 1 standard deviation indicated by the dotted lines. The AEV amplitudes measured from subject SG from Figure 3.14 are displayed as the solid squares.

Amplifier filter bandwidth effects

The AEVs must be measured using a wide amplifier bandwidth in order not to distort the waveforms. For our normative and clinical studies, we have consistently used 1–10,000 Hz as our recording bandwidth. However, to illustrate the effects of inadequate bandwidth for AEVs, we have measured the effects of systematically changing the amplifier bandwidth for two adult cochlear implant patients with complete insertion of all active electrodes and stiffening rings. These results are shown in Figure 3.17a with a fixed high frequency filter of 10,000 Hz in combination with low frequency (high-pass) settings of 0.01, 1, 5, 10, 30, 100, 150 and 300 Hz. In Figure 3.17b, we summarize the effects of systematically varying the amplifier bandwidth by leaving the low frequency (high-pass) filter at 1 Hz in combination with high frequency (low-pass) filter settings of 30, 100, 250, 500, 1,000, 1,500, 3,000 and 10,000 Hz. These results demonstrate that high frequency cut-offs of less than 3,000 Hz and low frequency cut-offs greater than 30 Hz will distort AEVs. These distortions include asymmetric biphasic AEVs and reduced peak-to-peak amplitudes. These results were obtained for a 200 µs/phase stimulus. The exact effect of bandwidth is dependent on the evoked potential system because of differences in filter configuration.

The AEV waveform distortion effects from lowering the high frequency filter and increasing the low frequency filter are illustrated in Figure 3.18. Significant distortion of the AEV waveforms can result from the use of reduced bandwidths, which make the AEVs appear to be 'abnormal'. The use

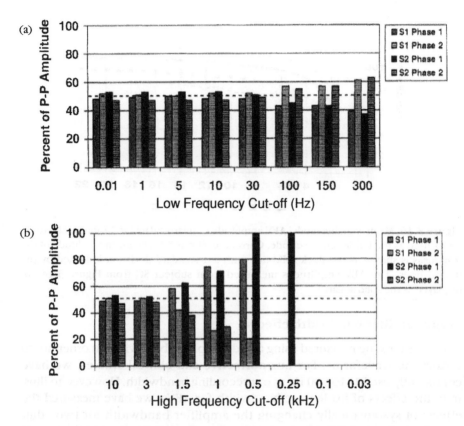

Figure 3.17. AEV amplitudes for waveform phases 1 and 2. Results are shown for two subjects (S1 and S2). Figure 17(a) the low cut-off frequency was varied from 0.01 to 300 Hz whereas the upper frequency was held constant at 10,000 Hz. Figure 17(b) the high frequency cut-off was varied from 10,000 Hz to 250 Hz as the low frequency cut-off was held constant at 1 Hz. These filter characteristics caused systematic changes in the phase 1 versus phase 2 asymmetry as illustrated in these summary graphs, especially when the high frequency cut-off was varied. Note the transition to monophasic responses at frequencies below 1,500 Hz.

of the 1 to 1,000 Hz bandwidth reduces the overall amplitude of the AEV (upper tracing) and causes significant phase distortion and amplitude reduction. The 100 to 10,000 Hz bandwidth produces an apparent differential effect between the two phases of the biphasic AEV (lower tracing) in comparison to the wide bandwidth (1 to 10,000 Hz) AEV shown in the centre tracing of Figure 3.18. We recommend that a wide bandwidth should always be used without the use of a 'notch-filter' to avoid effects of ringing due to the narrow bandpass filtering. Postmeasurement digital filters or

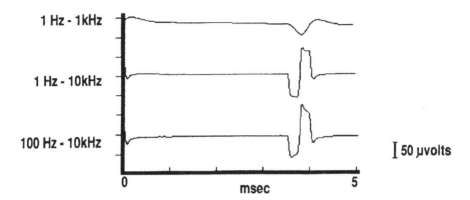

Figure 3.18. AEV waveforms for three frequency bandwidth conditions. The centre tracing is the reference bandwidth condition (1 to 10,000 Hz) used for all normative data obtained in our experiments. Note that the two phases of the AEV are essentially equal in amplitude and phase duration. The upper tracing shows the AEV pattern for the bandwidth of 1 to 1,000 Hz. Note the significant amplitude reduction and the phase shift (delay). In the lower tracing, the AEV for a 100 to 10,000 Hz bandwidth is shown. The two AEV phases are not equal in amplitude, which was illustrated in Figure 3.17(a) (100 Hz data points) where phase 1 has less amplitude than phase 2.

'smoothing' can be used to eliminate some interference signals selectively, but usually this is not necessary. We occasionally encounter high frequency interference when recording AEVs intraoperatively, which can be filtered out *post hoc*. In general, we avoid any *post hoc* data manipulations in preference to working with the original AEV waveforms.

Effects of averager sampling rate

Sampling rates must be high enough to resolve each phase of the biphasic AEVs in order to avoid distortion. The evoked potential system we used (Nicolet Compact Four) has 512 digital sampling points per sweep. In this instance, the sweep time should not exceed 25 ms in order not to violate the Nyqvist theorem. To illustrate the distortions possible from an inadequate sampling rate, we measured AEVs in 19 of our normative subjects using the following parameters: electrode 10 active, electrode 1 indifferent, pulse rate of 250 Hz, pulse width 204 µs/phase and a current level of 65 µA. The analysis window was then changed to measure AEV distortions. The analysis times included 10, 20, 30, 40, 50, 60 and 70 ms. As illustrated in Figure 3.19, undersampling results in asymmetric AEV waveform morphology and reduced peak-to-peak amplitudes. Based on these results, we recommend that the minimum sampling rate be set to satisfy the following constraint:

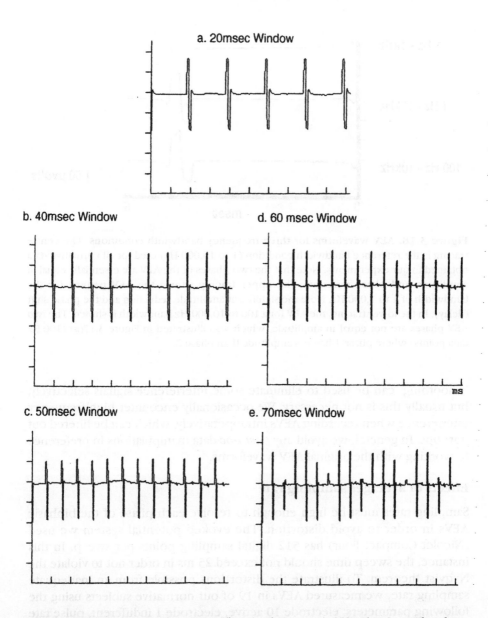

Figure 3.19. Sampling rate distortions. The stimulation rate is 250 pulses/second so that a pulse will occur every 4 ms. In panel 19a (20 ms) note that the responses are symmetrical and clearly resolved by the signal averager. The same result is observed for the analysis time window of 40 ms (19b). However from 50 ms (19c) to 70 ms (19e), there is an increasing distortion of the waveforms because the signal averaging does not adequately resolve these AEV waveforms.

$$\text{sampling rate} = \frac{\text{number of points/sweep}}{\text{time window}} \geq 2 \times \text{high frequency cut-off}$$

In general, to avoid these distortions we recommend minimum analysis times of 25 ms for 512 sampling points, 12 ms for 256 sampling points, and so forth. The sampling rate must be high enough to provide at least three data points for each phase of stimulation. With only one or two data points, the amplitude of AEV waveforms will often be distorted.

Adequate and consistent averager triggering

We use a TTL trigger from the Nucleus cochlear implant stimulation equipment to trigger our signal averager. When the DPI is set to 'Direct', the timing of the 5 V positive TTL pulse with respect to the biphasic stimulus is thus synchronized with the stimulus onset. It is not adequate simply to use the input preamplifier signal as the triggering signal. When this is done, inconsistent triggering of the signal averager will result in distorted AEV waveforms due to the 'jitter' associated with variations in the start time of averaging.

Recording electrode montages

Based on our unpublished preliminary investigations recording electrode voltages at 30 different sites on the scalp, we determined that the largest AEV measurement is obtained when using the ipsilateral mastoid as the positive electrode, vertex as the negative electrode and forehead as the ground electrode (montage A in Figure 3.2). In order to quantify the improvement in the signal levels achieved using this montage, AEVs were measured using montage A and the other more conventional montages, B and C (see Figure 3.2).

For each montage, the peak-to-peak AEV amplitude was normalized with respect to the peak-to-peak AEV amplitude measured for montage A. For the 19 subjects tested, the mean result for each montage is shown in Figure 3.20. These results demonstrate that montage A provides approximately a 10% increase in signal level above that obtained using montage B and approximately 20% increase in signal level above that obtained using montage C.

Effects of RF interference

The Nucleus 22 channel cochlear implant uses a 2.5 MHz RF carrier to transmit power and stimulation information to the internal receiver/stimulator. The RF carrier will vary among cochlear implant devices, but the principles are similar. This RF is always present during electrode activation but it

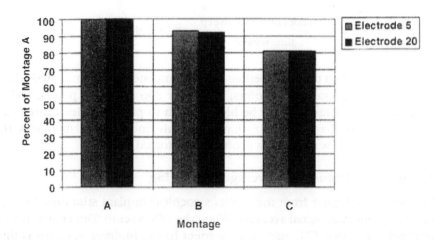

Figure 3.20. Normalized AEV amplitudes for the three electrode montages. All amplitudes are normalized to montage A as this montage produced the highest amplitudes of the AEVs. See Figure 3.2 for description of the three montages.

can be filtered out with a low-pass RF filter. However, if the RF filtering is not adequate, AEV recording can be contaminated. In cases where the measured AEVs are very small (<20 µV peak-to-peak), the RF artefact can obscure the AEVs completely. Some of these effects are shown in Figure 3.21, where tracing A represents a normal AEV without any RF interference. Tracing B in the same figure was obtained when the surface recording electrode leads were placed too close to the transmitting coil of the cochlear implant system. The lower tracing C in the figure demonstrates AEVs recorded without a RF filter. These RF distortions illustrated in Figure 3.21 were the two most common examples that we encountered during many hours of AEV recording sessions, however the morphology can vary widely. Based on our experience with the Nucleus 22 cochlear implant system, we recommend the AEV testing parameters that we list in Table 3.2. The parameters have been shown to minimize distorted AEV recordings and false interpretations.

The Crystal Integrity Test System

Overview

The Crystal Integrity Test System provides a way of quickly and easily performing a series of integrity checks on any Nucleus implant. For the Nucleus CI22M implant, AEVs are obtained under a variety of stimulus conditions, thus providing a data set that forms a comprehensive evaluation of most aspects of implant function. Some of the features of the Crystal produce

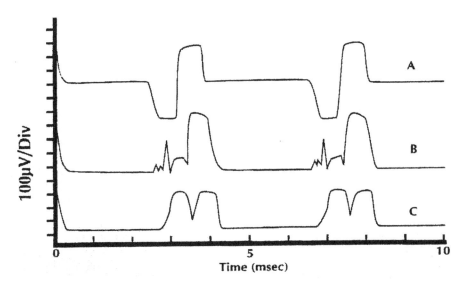

Figure 3.21. RF distortion of AEVs. The upper tracing (A) shows an AEV obtained without any significant RF interference. In B, we simply placed the AEV recording electrodes next to the headset transmitting coil during the recording. In C, the recordings were made without an effective low-pass RF filter.

Table 3.2. Recommended AEV protocol for the Nucleus 22 channel cochlear implants (CI22 and CI24). (Similar settings apply to other cochlear implant devices)

Electrode montage
Ipsilateral mastoid tip: (+) non-inverting amplifier input
Vertex: (–) inverting amplifier input
Forehead: amplifier ground

Recording amplifier and averager
Bandwidth: 1 to 10,000 Hz
RF filtering: 100 kHz low-pass
Gain: avoid clipping or under-amplification (120,000 or less)
Sampling rate: 20,000 Hz minimum
Time window adequate to resolve waveforms; e.g. 10 μs

Stimulation parameters
Bipolar mode with wide electrode spacing
Pulse widths ≥ 75 μs
Rate 200–300 Hz

results similar to the 'stimulogram' described by Almqvist et al. (1993). For the more recent Nucleus CI24 implant, the Crystal collects both AEV and telemetry data. An example of a stimulogram (provided by Almqvist) is shown in Figure 3.22. This example was obtained from a CI22M device in 'variable' mode where all active electrodes are paired to electrode 1 as the indifferent, which simulates a monopolar mode. His procedure was developed using a custom-built system and provides a quick way to scan the AEVs of a CI22M device.

The Crystal Integrity Test System is shown in Figure 3.23. It consists of a 'black box' containing the hardware necessary both to generate the RF signals that drive the implant, and to collect and amplify the AEV and telemetry information returned from the implant. The box also contains a storage compartment for the cables necessary for driving the implant, recording the AEV signals and communicating with the computer when the system is not in use. The system is controlled by software running on a laptop computer. The computer interfaces to the Crystal via the serial port (which controls the implant operation) and a data acquisition card plugged into the computer (which digitizes the returned AEV data).

Previous systems of this nature have been bulky and complicated to set up and operate. One of the design goals of the Crystal system was that with minimal training a cochlear implant clinician (not a company specialist) should be able to collect a standard set of data without assistance. The data are stored in a common file format so it can easily be e-mailed to a company representative for interpretation. The intention is that larger clinics will elect to keep a system available locally so that implant users can be tested as the need arises. This means that clinicians can have immediate access to an integrity test and can have an interpretation available within hours. At present, an integrity test typically involves arranging a visit from a company representative at a time that suits the recipient, the clinician and the company representative. This process can take days or even weeks to organize. As an integrity test is often the first step in diagnosing users who are reporting problems, the Crystal offers the prospect of significantly speeding up the diagnostic process and improving user care. Further information about the Crystal Integrity Test System can be obtained from Cochlear Limited.

System operation

The clinician controls Crystal through a Windows-based interface program that runs on a laptop computer. On starting the program an information screen appears and allows the user to enter information related to the user and the test. Certain information on this screen is mandatory and certain information is optional.

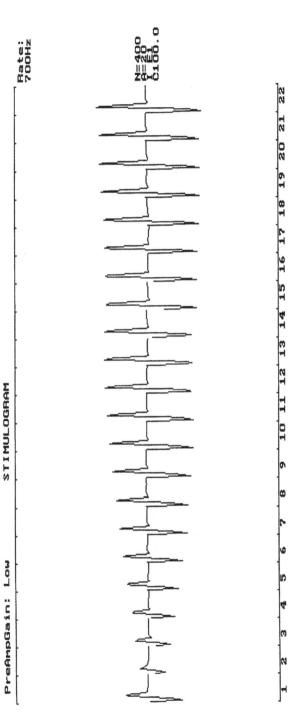

Figure 3.22. Example of a stimulogram. Provided by Bengt Almqvist, University Hospital in Lund, Sweden. This technique is incorporated into some of the tests performed with the Crystal Integrity Test System.

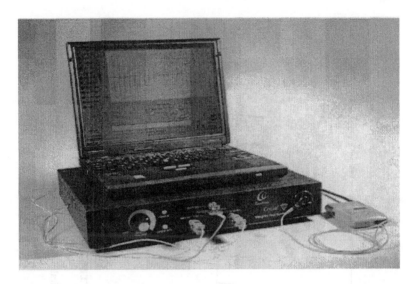

Figure 3.23. The Crystal Integrity Test System. It is a self-contained unit that operates efficiently with a laptop computer to objectively test the functioning of Nucleus CI22 or CI24 devices.

When all the mandatory information has been entered, the user may proceed to the test screen, which is where the bulk of the test is conducted. Figure 3.24 shows an example of the test screen. The list on the left side of the screen shows all the tests that are recommended for the particular type of implant that has been selected. This example shows the test screen from a Nucleus 22 device running the 'Current Level' test. Note that the list is tailored for the Nucleus 22 device and contains certain tests that would not appear if the device being tested were a Nucleus 24 device (such as the 'Pseudo MP' test). When a test has been performed and data from it have been saved, a check mark appears next to the test to indicate that it is complete.

AEV data are digitized by the system and is presented to the operator in an 'oscillograph' format on the screen. The relevant stimulation and recording parameters are all preset to default values so that in most cases all the operator has to do is to increase the current level until a clear signal is displayed. The display can be frozen — to allow close inspection of the captured signal — or saved, or both. In the lower section of the screen the clinician has control over certain aspects of the stimulation and recording parameters. Past experience has shown that when trying to record AEV data, even experienced clinicians can be easily confused when combinations of pulse width, rate and oscilloscope time base are arbitrarily varied. Interactions between the oscilloscope sampling rate and the pulsatile signal are notorious for giving false indications of absent or abnormal pulses for

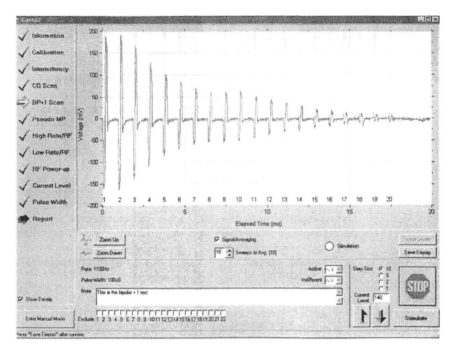

Figure 3.24. Main test screen of the Crystal. It displays an electrode scan using BP+1 mode with only 16 averages (sweeps). This main screen also displays the other tests that can be performed on the left side of the window.

example. Therefore these parameters are preset by Crystal to provide the optimum stimulus and recording conditions for each test and are deliberately not adjustable in this screen. The operator can control other parameters, which are not so likely to affect the interpretation of the test, such as the vertical zoom of the display or the number of averages used. For less experienced operators the 'show details' switch can be turned off and a more limited set of controls becomes available. This makes the display less intimidating and in most cases adequate recordings can be made with little or no change to the default values.

Tables 3.3 and 3.4 show lists of all the Crystal tests that are available for the Nucleus 22 and Nucleus 24 devices respectively and give a brief description of what the tests do and why they are performed. An important aspect of any integrity test system is the requirement that it must reliably self-calibrate. When trying to determine if an implant is faulty or not, it is essential to be able to check the integrity of the test system in order to conclude safely that any abnormal results are due to the implant and not to the integrity test system. To this end the Crystal system has a test implant built directly behind its front panel with a load network and a three-pin output designed to

Table 3.3. Crystal Tests for the Nucleus CI22M device

Name	Function	Purpose
Calibration	Provides a continuous pulse stream of moderate rate	To check the integrity of the test system, cables etc. This test is performed with the transmitter coil and recording electrodes connected to the built-in test implant behind the Crystal front panel
Intermittency	Provides a continuous pulse stream of moderate rate. The user is instructed to manipulate the implant site while observing the output waveform for any gaps or missed pulses	To check for intermittent behaviour of the implant. The intention behind manipulating the implant site is to try and uncover any latent problems with the implant which may be exacerbated by mechanical movement
Common Ground (CG) scan	Provides a single-shot series of pulses in CG mode scanning from electrodes 1 to 22 along the electrode array. All 22 pulses are presented simultaneously on the screen	
Bipolar + 1 (BP+1) scan	Provides a single-shot series of pulses in BP+1 mode from electrodes 1 to 20 along the electrode array. All 20 pulses are presented simultaneously on the screen	To help check for electrode shorts, opens or other anomalies in conjunction with the other two scan tests. May also be possible to infer the extent of certain cochlear pathologies from the overall shape of the scans
Pseudomonopolar (PseudoMP) scan	Provides a single-shot series of pulses in pseudomonopolar mode (1 to 2, 1 to 3 etc.) from electrodes 2 to 22 along the electrode array. All 21 pulses are presented simultaneously on the screen	
High rate/RF	Provides a continuous pulse stream near the *maximum* rate for the implant. The amplitude of the transmitted RF is varied by the user during this test	Checks for implant function at or near its *maximum* rate. Since the implant is powered from the transmitted RF, the RF level is varied to determine if implant operation is affected by this
Low rate/RF	Provides a continuous pulse stream near the *minimum* rate for the implant. The amplitude	Checks for implant function at or near its *minimum* rate. Since the implant is powered from the

Table 3.3. (cont'd)

Name	Function	Purpose
	of the transmitted RF is varied by the user during this test	transmitted RF, the RF level is reduced to determine if the implant continues to function at combinations of low rate and low RF level
RF Power-up	Provides a single-shot burst of moderate rate pulses with no preceding power-up pulses. The recording is triggered to coincide with the beginning of the pulse train. The first few pulses on the display are therefore missing because the device takes a few pulses before it becomes powered and can output stimulation	To check that the device can power up in a normal amount of time. Problems with the power management circuitry or integrated circuit power supply requirements are indicated if the device takes longer than normal to power up
Current level	Provides a single shot train of pulses where the current level increases from zero to a maximum value set by the user and then ramps down again in a series of steps	To check whether the implant can output stimulation pulses at varying current levels as programmed by the system
Pulse width	Provides a single shot series of pulses where the pulse width increases from 25 to 500 µs in a series of steps	To check whether the implant can output stimulation pulses at varying pulse widths as programmed by the system

simulate the output obtained from a recipient. The first test in any series is always calibration, which is performed on the test implant to ensure the integrity of the system. When this is successfully completed, the RF transmission cable and the AEV recording electrodes are transferred to the recipient and the implant test is performed. Often the calibration test is repeated after the implant test as further confirmation of correct test system function.

Experienced clinicians wishing to control further aspects of the stimulation and recording arbitrarily can enter the Manual Mode screen. Figure 3.25 shows an example of the Manual Mode screen. In this screen, features such as high- and low-pass filter adjustment (achieved by electronic control of hardware filters), and RF power control are available. In addition, Manual Mode allows the control of other parameters that may be fixed in many of the

Table 3.4. Crystal Tests for the Nucleus CI24 device

The tests available are as featured in Table 3.3, with the following additional procedures.

Name	Function	Purpose
Telemetry	Records voltages on all electrodes during a preset stimulus sequence in common ground mode and returns the data via implant back telemetry	Reliably checks all electrodes for opens and shorts and checks for correct operation of the implant telemetry system
Monopolar 1 (MP1) Scan	Provides a single-shot series of pulses in monopolar 1 mode (to the ball extracochlear electrode) scanning from electrodes 1 to 22 along the electrode array. All 22 pulses are presented simultaneously on the screen	To help check for intracochlear electrode shorts and opens and the integrity of the MP1 and MP2 extracochlear electrodes respectively. May also be possible to infer the extent of certain cochlear pathologies from the overall shape of the scans
Monopolar 2 (MP2) Scan	Provides a single-shot series of pulses in monopolar 2 mode (to the plate extracochlear electrode) scanning from electrodes 1 to 22 along the electrode array. All 22 pulses are presented simultaneously on the screen	

tests. One further feature of this screen is 'Live Speech' mode where the oscilloscope is set into a free running (non-triggered) mode and no stimulation is provided by the Crystal system. Here a separate processor can be used to drive the recipient's implant and the resulting pulses can be viewed on the screen. This is particularly useful when diagnosing problems that may result from an interaction between the user's external processor and the implant.

Finally, the program allows users to review waveforms that have been saved during the test. In the Report screen, waveforms can be inspected more closely using the vertical and horizontal zoom feature, notes can be modified or appended as desired and the waveforms can be deleted if no longer required. All the parameter information associated with each recorded waveform is also displayed.

Application of Crystal measurements

Crystal is effective in diagnosing most common faults found in cochlear implants. Many faults, such as the complete absence of stimulation current

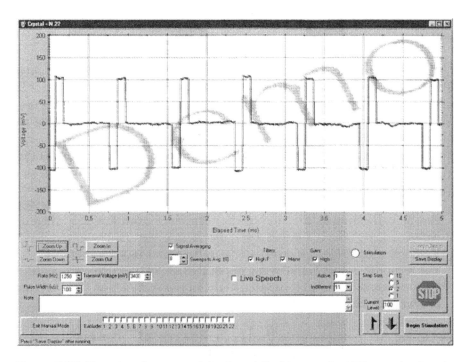

Figure 3.25. Manual mode screen of the Crystal. In this case, the AEVs to a simple pulse series are displayed for one electrode of a Nucleus 22 device. Note that the AEV amplitudes are consistent and appear to be stable.

due to a failed internal component, are easy to confirm by the absence or unusual nature of the recorded AEVs. Electrode short and open circuits are particularly amenable to diagnosis using the scan tests. In a scan test, stimulation is programmed from different electrodes on the intracochlear array with the electrode position scanned from one end of the array to the other. For electrode arrays with no short or open circuits, a distinctive overall shape to the envelope formed by the stimulus pulses can be seen. No sudden changes in AEV amplitude or phase occur between adjacent electrodes. Crystal uses scan tests that operate in three different stimulation modes (for Nucleus 22 devices common ground, BP+1 and pseudomonopolar modes) because each mode reacts differently to a fault. By comparing results from all three scan tests, it is often possible to be confident of the nature of a fault that may remain ambiguous following a scan in a single mode. Some scan results show abrupt changes in amplitude from electrode to electrode that are not consistent with scans from other modes. In these cases there is probably some factor other than electrode short and open circuits influencing the AEV amplitudes (for example, unusual cochlear structure) and it may well not be a fault with the electrode array.

The following factors govern the phase and amplitude of an AEV response in a healthy cochlea:

- The response amplitude increases monotonically with the distance between the active and indifferent stimulating electrodes.
- The phase of the response is governed by the direction of current flow along the cochlear duct. Apical to basal flow gives the opposite phase to basal to apical flow.
- The response amplitude decreases monotonically with the distance of the stimulating electrode pair from the base of the cochlea, in a bipolar mode.
- Where more than one active or reference electrode exists (for example, common ground mode or if electrodes are shorted) response amplitudes can be calculated as the sum of the responses from multiple current paths.
- Response amplitudes are proportional to the stimulation current.
- The response is unaffected by the physical shape of the cochlear duct (the cochlea could be straight, or spiral in the opposite direction and the scan test would look the same).

Diagnosing electrode problems then becomes a case of comparing the AEVs produced from a particular implant with the expected 'normal' result. One other area of interest arises from a study of the scan test implemented in the Crystal. A small percentage of recipients have scans that show the AEV amplitudes undulating, as if the amplitude were modulated by the physical direction of the electrode array with respect to the recording electrodes. This might be expected if segments of the bone of the cochlea were electrically more conductive. Then the dipole created by stimulation in a bipolar mode would indeed be very dependent on the physical orientation of the stimulating electrodes as well as the recording electrodes. Some users with these types of scan results have had otosclerosis, a condition know to produce porous bone, as we have shown for patient DW (Figures 3.8 and 3.9). While there is no direct evidence as yet that an undulating scan test is indicative of porous bone in the cochlea it would seem to be an area worthy of further study. If it indeed is the case, then it may be that Crystal scans could prove to be a useful tool in diagnosing and tracking the progress of the disease.

The Crystal Integrity Test System is a new and clinically useful tool for diagnosing implant faults of various kinds. It relies on AEVs recorded using a variety of stimulation and recording conditions for diagnosing Nucleus products. For Nucleus 24 implants, a combination of AEVs and telemetry are used. It may also prove useful in diagnosing and monitoring cochlear pathologies such as otosclerosis and meningitis that change the electrical resistance of the cochlear structures. Its ease of use makes it possible for cochlear implant clinicians, not just specialized company representatives, to perform the various tests. This means that integrity testing can be performed much more routinely than in the past, hopefully improving the level of care for cochlear implant users.

Discussion

We have refined the testing methods that can be used to verify the integrity of the internal components of the Nucleus standard and Mini-22 cochlear implants and the Nucleus 24 devices. The AEVs are measured from stimulation at 250 Hz, typically at a constant current of approximately 300 μA in BP+1 and at 65 μA for the wide bipolar modes. In BP+1, the AEV amplitudes varied from 200 μV peak-to-peak on the basal electrodes down to less than 10 μV peak-to-peak from the apical electrodes (Figure 3.6). When we used electrode 1 as the indifferent electrode (pseudomonopolar) for increasingly wider bipolar modes from base to apex, the AEV amplitudes increased proportionally with the increasing width of the stimulation modes (BP to BP+20). Using this technique, the group averages for normally functioning devices ranged from 20 μV peak-to-peak for basal electrode 2 to about 130 μV peak-to-peak for apical electrode 22 (Figure 3.16). The AEV amplitudes from the apical electrodes are significantly larger in these modes at a stimulation current of 65 μA, in comparison to the AEV values of the apical electrodes obtained in BP+1 at a current of 300 μA. In the latter case, the AEVs averaged less than 20 μV for the same apical electrodes (Figure 3.6). Averaged electrode voltages measured using widening bipolar modes result in larger AEV peak-to-peak amplitudes as the active electrode moves more apically, and a more consistent trend of increasing AEV amplitude with increase in distance between the active and indifferent electrode in the normal cochlea. For these reasons, we now prefer to use the wider bipolar modes for the measurement of AEVs rather than BP+1 (Shallop, 1993b; Shipp et al., 1993; Mahoney and Rotz Proctor, 1994) or common ground as recommended by Kileny et al. (1995). We do *not* recommend the use of common ground for AEV measurements because of the distortions that can result, as demonstrated in Figures 3.10, 3.11, 3.12 and 3.13.

Signal averaging with a clinical evoked potential system or the Crystal Integrity Test System enhances the reliability of detecting responses on all usable electrodes. We can also monitor the real time amplified (un-averaged) waveforms and the audio output of the amplifier to observe the consistency of the AEVs across the electrode array. This enables us to check for intermittent AEVs, which could be an indication of electrode array or receiver stimulator problems.

In narrow bipolar (BP or BP+1) and common ground modes, the observed AEV waveforms were always phase leading negative to positive in the basal turn, and in some patients phase reversal of the waveforms was observed as the measurement sequence moved toward the apex of the cochlea. With the technique of using electrode 1 as a constant indifferent electrode, we have never observed phase reversals or asymmetric phase amplitudes in 'normal' cases. The two forms of distortion (phase reversal and decreased AEV amplitudes) were often observed in narrow bipolar and common ground modes, typically from middle or apical electrodes of the array. The phase reversals are most likely due to the location and orientation of the stimulation dipole relative to the plane of the recording electrodes. The volume conduction from the electrode array to the surface electrodes must also have an effect on the measured AEVs, especially in common ground where the direction of current flow is less predictable.

The BP+1 AEV results of 30 adult patients have been analysed and can be used as normative data for comparison purposes either in BP+1 (see Figure 3.6) as reported by Peterson et al. (1995) or in varied wide pseudomonopolar bipolar modes (see Figures 3.14 to 3.16). These mean response amplitudes (± 1 SD) by electrode number thus provide a way to display and compare results from specific cases. We recommend AEV measurements using a device such as the Crystal system for a time-efficient technique to verify device and electrode function. The AEV measures also provide a method to make long-term comparisons in specific patients over extended postoperative time periods. These techniques have been shown to be especially useful with paediatric patients (Mahoney and Rotz Proctor, 1995) or with any patient when the functioning of the internal device or specific electrodes needs to be evaluated (Kileny et al., 1995; Peterson et al., 1995). The reader is cautioned that the ± 1 standard deviation results (Figures 3.6 and 3.16) should not be used as delineation between normal and abnormal implant function.

The possibility of AEV waveform distortion is more likely when narrow pulse widths are used in combination with high rates of stimulation. This result is likely in the techniques used by Mens et al. (1993; 1994a; 1994b) and by Almqvist et al. (1993) if the signal averager does not have adequate sampling rates. These authors typically used time analysis epochs of 50–75 ms, which may not adequately resolve AEV waveforms with pulse widths of 200 μs or less. Although the electrode-by-electrode mapping technique of Mens and colleagues, and the stimulogram technique of Almqvist et al. provide a quick way to assess all of the electrodes, we prefer to make certain that we have adequate resolution of the waveforms through the combination of sampling rate and time analysis window. This clearly resolves AEV waveforms, as demonstrated in the Crystal electrode scans.

An example of AEVs recorded from a CLARION cochlear implant with pulse widths of 75, 150 and 300 μs/phase is shown in Figure 3.26. The stimulation rate is 200 pulses per second. The specific analysis parameters for

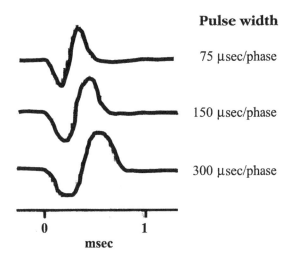

Pulse width

75 µsec/phase

150 µsec/phase

300 µsec/phase

0   1

msec

Figure 3.26. AEV recordings from a CLARION cochlear implant. Provided by Phil Segel, Advanced Bionics Corporation. Note that there is a reduction in amplitude for the 75 µs/phase AEVs in comparison with the 150 and 300 µs/phase AEVs. The CLARION system AEV set-up parameters are detailed in Appendix 3.2.

these recordings are not known, but they illustrate the need to use valid acquisition parameters in order to resolve the true waveforms. In this illustration, the amplitude of the 75 µs waveform is slightly reduced in comparison to the amplitudes of the 150 and 300 µs waveforms.

We have also demonstrated the need to record AEVs with wide band filters (1 to 10,000 Hz) and the proper amplifier gain in order to obtain optimal recordings without distortion of the biphasic waveforms. When the high-pass filter is moved upward or the low-pass filter is moved downward, distorted AEV waveforms will result. AEVs measured with restricted bandwidth do not provide an accurate measure of the output from a cochlear implant and can lead to misinterpretation of the results. Improper selection of preamplifier gain can cause clipped waveforms with over-amplification and poor resolution when the amplifier gain is too small. Optimal settings need to be established with specific equipment, but we recommend that the preamplifier sensitivity should be set initially to 1,000 µV (gain = 120,000) and adjusted as needed to optimize the AEV waveforms. We recommend that acquisition parameters be selected carefully in order to avoid the need to perform offline operations in an attempt to optimize recordings as suggested by Mens et al. (1994a).

Originally, we recommended that the recording electrode montage should be ipsilateral to contralateral mastoid with a ground on the forehead

(Heller et al., 1991). However, we now know that AEV amplitudes will be the largest when they are recorded using the ipsilateral mastoid and the vertex (Cz) as the two active electrodes (montage A in Figure 3.2).

Based on our findings and those of other authors cited throughout this chapter, we recommend the protocol listed in Table 3.2 for obtaining AEVs with the Nucleus 22 channel cochlear implant. This protocol has evolved from our research and clinical testing with more than 100 cochlear implant patients as well as laboratory 'tank tests'. For specific recommended proce-dures for the Nucleus and CLARION devices, see Appendices 3.1 and 3.2 respectively.

Conclusions

Averaged electrode voltages provide a time-efficient method to verify the integrity of the internal components of a multichannel cochlear implant. A clinical evoked potential system can be used to obtain responses at small voltages below that which can typically be measured by real time oscillo-scope techniques without signal averaging. The external triggering of an oscilloscope or an evoked potential system must be of adequate voltage and consistent timing such as a TTL pulse. If triggering is reliable, it is less likely that AEV waveforms will be distorted by time jitter or missed pulses from the cochlear implant.

Averaged electrode voltage measurements and telemetry can be used with children and adults as a postoperative test whenever device or electrode failure is suspected. It is also possible to use the procedure intraoperatively during flap closure because all electrodes can be tested in a few minutes. We also suggest that the preamplifier signal be monitored via an audio output and real time 'input' signal to the averager as additional verification of device and electrode function. AEV recordings can easily be distorted by the RF transmission signal, which carries the data pulses from the speech processor to the internal receiver stimulator. It is important to carefully route recording electrode leads away from the transmitting coil and use a RF filter to minimize RF contamination of AEVs. AEVs can also be distorted significantly by using common ground mode, limited preamplifier bandwidth or inadequate analogue to digital sampling rates.

Acknowledgements

The authors wish to thank the many cochlear implant patients who volun-teered their time to help us obtain the data we present in this chapter. We give a special acknowledgement to Jim Heller, MSEE of Rela Corporation in

Boulder, Colorado. Jim was the project development engineer for the Crystal Integrity Test system, and formerly Director of Research Engineering at Cochlear Corporation. We also received the support and advice of other Cochlear engineers in Australia (David Money and Jim Patrick) and Switzerland (Ernst von Wallenberg). Thanks also to Phil Segel of Advanced Bionics Corporation for providing CLARION AEV tracings.

References

Almqvist B, Harris S, Jonsson KE (1993) The stimulogram. In Hochmair-Desoyer IJ, Hochmair ES (eds) Advances in Cochlear Implants. Wein: Manz, pp. 33–6.

Crosby PA, Seligman PM, Patrick JF, Kuzma JA, Money DK, Ridler J, Dowell R (1984) The Nucleus multi-channel implantable hearing prosthesis. Acta Otolaryngol Suppl (Stockh) 411: 111–14.

Heller JW, Shallop JK, Abbas PJ (1993) Cochlear implant assessment by averaged electrode voltages. In Hochmair-Desoyer IJ, Hochmair ES (eds) Advances in Cochlear Implants. Wein: Manz, pp. 255–9.

Heller JW, Sinopoli T, Fowler-Brehm N, Shallop JK (1991) The characterization of averaged electrode voltages from the Nucleus cochlear implant. IEEE Trans, November.

Kileny PR, Meiteles LZ, Zwolan TA, Telian SA (1995) Cochlear implant device failure: diagnosis and management. Am J Otol 16(2): 164–71.

Mahoney MJ, Rotz Proctor LA (1994) The use of averaged electrode voltages to assess the function of Nucleus internal cochlear implant devices in children. Ear Hear 15: 177–83.

Mens HM, Oostendorp T, Van den Broek P (1993) Electrode-by-electrode mapping of cochlear implant generated surface potentials: (partial) device failures. In Fraysse B, Deguine O (eds) Cochlear implants: new perspectives. Adv Otorhinolaryngol 48. Basel, Switzerland: Karger, pp. 75–8.

Mens HM, Oostendorp T, Van den Broek P (1994a) Identifying electrode failures with cochlear implant generated surface potentials. Ear Hear 15: 330–8.

Mens HM, Oostendorp T, Van den Broek P (1994b) Cochlear implant generated surface potentials: current spread and side effects. Ear Hear 15: 339–45.

Peterson AM, Bray RH, Facer GW (1995) Averaged electrode voltages used to identify nonfunctioning electrodes in cochlear implants: case study. J Am Acad Audiol 6: 243–9.

Shallop JK (1993a) Objective electrophysiological measures from cochlear implant patients. In Hochmair-Desoyer IJ, Hochmair ES (eds) Advances in Cochlear Implants. Wein: Manz, pp. 21–5.

Shallop JK (1993b) Objective electrophysiological measures from cochlear implant patients. Ear Hear 14: 58–63.

Shallop JK, Kelsall DC, Turnacliff KA (1993) Multichannel cochlear implant in children with labyrinthitis. In Hochmair-Desoyer IJ, Hochmair ES (eds) Advances in Cochlear Implants. Wein: Manz, pp. 470–3.

Shipp DB, Murad C, Nedzelski JM (1993) Test–retest reliability of averaged electrode voltage measurements with the Nucleus 22-Channel cochlear implant. In Hochmair-Desoyer IJ, Hochmair ES (eds) Advances in Cochlear Implants. Wein: Manz, pp. 252–4.

Appendix 3.1
Procedures for measuring AEVs from the Nucleus CI22 and CI24 cochlear implants

(Equipment used: Nicolet Compact Four/Auditory)

Compact Four settings

Modify set-up menu (status) as follows:
SEN = 1 K (Signal is very large, you may need to go higher)
LFF = 1 Hz, HFF = 10 kHz, *TRG = EXT, TME = 10 (5 for CI24),
SWP = 200 or less as needed.
The instructions for the Nicolet Compact systems can be used to guide the set-up of other evoked potential systems. The system used must have external trigger input enabled.
*Note: the CI22 trigger input is from the DPI audiologist headset jack using the cable available from Cochlear Limited. The CI24 interface card (IF5) has a standard BNC male trigger output connector that can easily be linked to the trigger input of the Compact 4.

AEV recording electrodes

+ Mastoid, Implant side
− Cz
GRND FPz

DPS v 6.100+ settings (F9)

Mode 'variable'
Rate 250 Hz
Keyboard duration 1,000 ms
Interstimulus 1 ms

DPS version 6.100+ settings (F3)

Electrodes 2–22 Active, PW = 200, CL = 50
(Equals about 65 μA)
Use electrode 1 as indifferent

Use G (Go) DPS command to stimulate. The stimulation rate is 250 Hz and the averaging will be very fast. Start the C4 averaging first and it will wait until you issue the G command to the implant. Use Memory 1 for electrode 2, M2 for electrode 3 and so forth. Store the first eight electrodes as files E2-9, then

E10–17 and E18–22. The testing takes about 5 minutes or less as you become familiar with the sequences. You can practise all of this in advance. If you use Apex files, a simple program can be written to expedite the averaging.

On the basal electrodes (2–8), the responses will be small but increasing in size (20–80 μV). If the averager is rejecting too much, decrease the sensitivity (increase numerically from 1K to 5K, and so on). After obtaining responses from electrodes 2 to 8 the responses will usually be 100–150 μV ± 75 μV and the sensitivity of the preamp can be adjusted as needed.

WIN-DPS R116 settings

Electrodes 1–22 Active, PW = 50, CL = 50
(Equals about 65 μA)
Use electrode MP1 as indifferent.

1. Run the WIN-Config program and enable the EABR trigger output.
2. Run the WIN-DPS program and create an ACE™ map to access all active electrodes. Select 'Preferences' to enable the EABR mode. Set the stimulation 'on' time to 1,000 ms and the interval to 1 ms. Set the 'start-up' pulses to begin at 1 ms longer than the analysis time window. For a 5 ms time analysis window, set this value to 6 ms. This ensures that the analysis window will not be contaminated with implant instruction pulses that will be superimposed on the EABR tracings.
3. Use the G (for example 999 G) command to initiate stimulation at appropriate levels. You can assure yourself that CL = 50 is *not* too loud for patients using appropriate psychophysical procedures. Next present the stimuli to acquire and store the AEV tracings.
4. Follow the additional suggestions above for DPS procedures.

The measured waveforms will be biphasic; negative followed by positive. With the electrode montage used, negative is displayed upward. Phase reversal and 'nulls' should not occur with the use of electrode 1 as fixed indifferent. Measure the peak-to-peak amplitude from each electrode and plot the results on a normative graph if available.

These suggestions are written for the Cochlear CI22 and CI24 devices. Similar procedures should enable clinicians to obtain AEVs from other cochlear implant devices. Contact the respective cochlear implant companies for specific instructions.

Appendix 3.2
Procedures for measuring averaged electrode voltages from the CLARION 1.2 and CII cochlear implants

(Equipment used: Nicolet Compact Four/Auditory)

Compact Four settings

Modify set-up menu (status) as follows:

SEN = 1K (Signal is very large, you may need to go higher)

LFF = 1 Hz, HFF = 10 kHz, *TRG = EXT, TME = 15,

SWP = 200 or less as needed

*Note: the CLARION TTL trigger output is from the Clinical Programming Interface, which has a standard BNC connector on the back. This output trigger should be connected to an evoked potential system or an oscilloscope via a cable to the external input of these devices.

AEV recording electrodes

+ Mastoid, Implant side

– Cz

GRND FPz

CLARION SCLIN 2000 settings

1. Create a patient file.
2. Right click on 'Measurements', pulsatile.
3. Select 'New' and EABR.
4. Select first electrode.
5. Leave polarity at 'normal' (negative-leading).
6. Set pulse rate to 100 Hz (maximum).
7. Set pulse width to 225 μs (pulse width default is 75 μs).
8. Set current level to 50 or desired level. Caution: the EABR mode is a monopolar mode. Be careful with levels when the patient is awake.
9. Since the maximum rate is 100 Hz in this version of SCLIN in the EABR mode, set the analysis time of the signal averager to 15 ms in order to see a clear AEV at 10 ms in this time window.
10. Stimulate and record AEVs on all electrodes. Use the evoked potential commands described in Appendix 3.1 to record and store AEVs.

These suggestions are written for the Advanced Bionics Corporation CLARION 1.2 and CII cochlear implant devices. Similar procedures should enable clinicians to obtain AEVs from other cochlear implant devices. Contact the respective cochlear implant companies for specific instructions.

Chapter 4

Electrically evoked stapedial reflexes: utility in cochlear implant patients

Annelle V Hodges, Stacy L Butts, John E King

Contents

Introduction

As discussed in Chapter 1, effective programming is vital in order to provide maximum benefit for cochlear implant patients. In our department, electrically evoked stapedial reflex thresholds (ESRTs) are used extensively in both adults and children. This chapter will describe the methods and clinical use of reflex measurements in the Nucleus®, CLARION® and MED-EL cochlear implant systems; unfortunately we do not have experience with the MXM device.

As early as 1986, clinical researchers determined that electrical stimulation of the auditory system could result in measurable contraction of the stapedius muscle in a manner similar to measurement of the acoustic stapedial reflex (Jerger et al., 1986; Jerger et al., 1988). The stapedial reflex, whether acoustically or electrically evoked, is a neuromuscular reflex mediated through the brainstem. The afferent limb is the cochlear nerve. The efferent limb is both crossed and uncrossed. Both efferent limbs travel along the facial nerve to the stapedius muscle evoking a contraction following adequately intense stimulation of the peripheral auditory system. Contraction of the stapedius muscle moves the stapes, resulting in stiffening of the ossicular chain and reduced compliance of the middle ear system. The change in compliance can easily be measured and recorded with commercially available

81

immittance testing equipment. The acoustic and electrically evoked stapedial reflexes are essentially identical physiologically and anatomically. Both have a threshold and demonstrate amplitude growth to a point of saturation. Measurement techniques are also essentially identical, with recording of the response possible either ipsilaterally or contralaterally relative to the stimulated ear. Only the eliciting stimulus differs.

Literature review

Numerous reports have documented measurement of the electrically evoked stapedial reflex both intraoperatively and postoperatively.

Postoperative measures

The first report on electrically evoked stapedial reflex measures in humans presented data on a single Nucleus multichannel implant user, obtained after several months of implant use (Jerger et al., 1986). The researchers showed that the stapedial reflex could be elicited by electrical stimulation using a reflex averaging technique. Reflexes were obtained from activation of one medial, one apical and one basal electrode pair using three different bipolar modes. Results showed that the latency-intensity function of the electrically evoked reflex is similar to the acoustically elicited reflex, but differs in morphology and amplitude growth. No reflexes could be recorded in a second subject implanted with the same device.

This report was followed by a second (Jerger et al., 1988) in which ESRTs were found to correspond most closely to the preferred listening level of seven experienced Nucleus 22 implant users. Among these implant users, saturation of reflex amplitude growth occurred below the behaviourally perceived level of uncomfortable loudness. The authors suggest that the reflex growth function may be useful as a guideline for initial programming, particularly in young children.

Similar results were reported using the Vienna device (Stephan et al., 1988, 1990, 1991). In one study, stapedial reflexes were obtained in 10 out of 12 Vienna device users (Stephan et al., 1988). Seven of the subjects had intracochlear electrodes while the remaining five had extracochlear electrodes. Rather than the pulsatile stimulation used by the Nucleus device, these reflexes were elicited in response to sinusoidal stimuli. Reflexes were obtained equally in both intracochlear and extracochlear electrode users. Reflex threshold was found to occur consistently between the most comfortable listening level and the level of loudness discomfort. A follow-up report (Stephan et al., 1991) again showed good agreement between the reflex threshold and the upper portion of the comfortable listening range, although the percentage of patients displaying reflexes was much smaller.

In the largest series reported to date, Battmer et al. (1990) reported on a group of 25 experienced Nucleus 22 implant users, 19 of whom had measurable ESRTs. Like the previous studies, reflex thresholds were elicited at levels of approximately 70% to 80% of the listener's dynamic range, thus being most closely related to levels of maximum stimulation.

Several additional studies published over the last few years have repeatedly supported the relationship of the stapedial reflex to maximum comfortable loudness levels in cochlear implant users (Spivak and Chute, 1994a and 1994b; Van den Borne et al., 1994; Shallop and Ash, 1996; Hodges et al., 1997; Hodges et al., 1999; Hodges et al., 2000). Only slight differences were found in the strength of the relationship among basal (r = 0.85), medial (r = 0.92), or apical (r = 0.91) electrodes (Hodges et al., 1997). These studies were all in general agreement that reflexes could be obtained in approximately 65% of adult implant users. Spivak and Chute (1994b) and Hodges et al. (1997) both reported on the performance of patients using maps in which the maximum comfortable listening level (C level) was set at reflex threshold. In both studies, patients were found to perform at least as well if not slightly better using the reflex based maps. In addition, patients generally reported that the reflex map had an improved sound quality compared to their behaviourally set C level maps. It is also important to note that in the group of adult patients, all reflex thresholds occurred below the level of discomfort (Hodges et al., 1997).

Spivak and Chute (1994a) and Hodges and colleagues (Hodges et al., 1997, 1999) reported on reflex measurement in paediatric subjects using Nucleus 22 or CLARION cochlear implants. Reflexes were obtained in 63% (Spivak and Chute, 1994a) and 75% (Hodges et al., 1997) of children using the Nucleus 22; 65% of children using the CLARION showed reflexes (Hodges et al., 1999). In all cases, ossification of the cochlea related to meningitis was found to be the most common factor associated with lack of a reflex in the children. All paediatric Nucleus users with present reflexes had their C levels raised gradually to reflex threshold. All were reported to be wearing their device comfortably.

Hodges et al. (2000) obtained reflexes in 67% of Nucleus 24 adults and 83% of Nucleus 24 paediatric users. Again, the relationship between ESRT and the behavioural perception of maximum comfortable listening was very strong, with an r-value of 0.94 for the experienced adult users. This relationship is illustrated in Figure 4.1. In this study, the efficacy of stapedial reflexes was compared to current data on neural response telemetry (NRT™) (Brown et al., 2000; Hughes et al., 2000). It was concluded that stapedial reflexes provide a quicker, more precise estimate of maximal stimulation levels than does the current generation of NRT.

Finally, Butts et al. (2001) reported on the measurement of stapedial reflexes in both adult and paediatric MED-EL users. Regression analysis

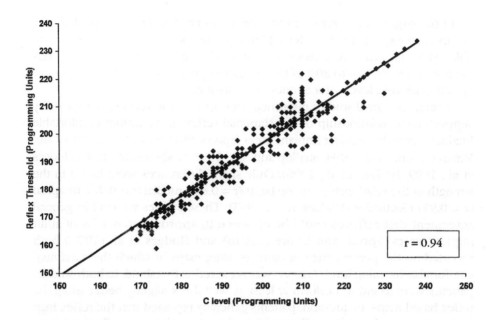

Figure 4.1. Relationship between C levels and ESRTs in postlingually deafened adult Nucleus 24 users.

confirmed a strong predictive relationship between ESRT and the most comfortable listening level (MCL) in adult MED-EL users. All reflex thresholds were obtained below the level of discomfort. Figure 4.2 is the scatterplot illustrating this relationship. Examples of reflexes obtained at different pulse durations from a MED-EL user are shown in Figure 4.3.

In each of these investigations, ESRTs have been evaluated as a means of estimating levels of current, either minimum or maximum, appropriate for CI users. Hodges et al. (1996) addressed reflexes in relation to another aspect of programming, that of loudness balancing. Experienced postlingually deafened adult implant users consistently judged current levels set at reflex threshold to be of equal loudness. In most cases, loudness balancing is not attempted with children. Further study is warranted, but if equal loudness balance can be consistently achieved with reflexes, the benefit is obvious.

Intraoperative measures

Several researchers have also looked at the viability and functional use of intraoperative reflex measurements. In children who may be unable to sit quietly for reflex testing during programming, or in children who are prone to recurrent middle-ear disease, obtaining reflex information while the child is anaesthetized for surgery may offer a viable option. Van den Borne et al. (1996) reported on a group of 19 children implanted with the Nucleus 22 in

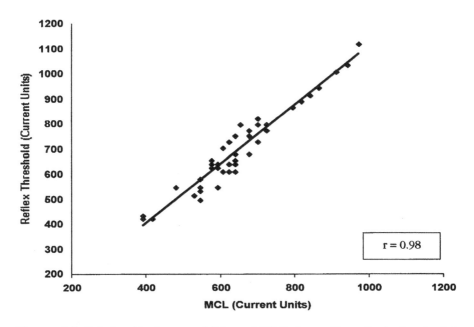

Figure 4.2. Relationship between MCLs and ESRTs in postlingually deafened adult MED-EL users.

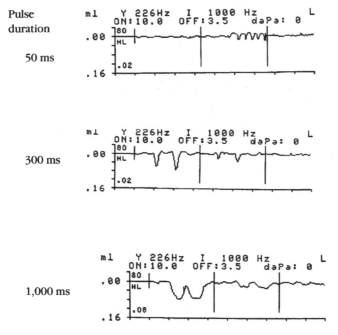

Figure 4.3. Examples of ESRTs obtained from a MED-EL user. Each panel shows the reflex obtained with a different pulse duration.

whom reflex measurements were made following insertion of the electrode array, prior to closing the incision. The transmitter coil was placed into a sterile plastic bag for positioning over the receiver-stimulator. Stimuli were presented via the Diagnostic Programming Interface, just as is done during postoperative programming. The presence of a reflex was judged based on visual detection of the stapedius muscle contraction. Reflexes were present in 79% of the children, and like the other studies, cochlear ossification related to meningitis was most often associated with absence of the reflex. Reflexes measured in this manner were found to be an average of 44 Nucleus programming units above the behavioural indication of C level obtained during later device programming. Taking into account the effects of anaesthetic agents, the researchers proposed a 'correction factor'. By applying the correction factor, adjusted intraoperatively measured reflexes were still found to be an average of 18 Nucleus programming units higher than behaviourally determined C levels. These particular researchers concluded that intraoperative stapedial reflex measurements have limited value in device fitting.

Two additional studies concluded that intraoperative stapedial reflex measurements are easy to make, and are useful in postoperative device-fitting procedures (Lindstrom and Bredberg, 1997; Opie et al., 1997). Lindstrom and Bredberg reported that a reflex could be visualized in each of 18 children evaluated during surgery. Opie and colleagues were able to obtain reflex measures in patients receiving CLARION, Nucleus and MED-EL devices during intraoperative procedures.

Makhdoum and colleagues (1998) looked more specifically at the effects of volatile anaesthetics on ESRTs. They too applied a correction factor to account for the increase in reflex thresholds due to anaesthetic agents. Although their corrected results were quite similar to those reported by Van den Borne et al. (1996), their conclusions regarding the utility of intraoperative stapedial reflex measures were more positive.

Almquist et al. (2000) reported on a procedure for measuring averaged stapedius muscle reflexes intraoperatively. During surgery, an EMG recording electrode was placed directly into the stapedius muscle. After placement of the electrode array, stimuli were presented via the transmitting coil by a custom designed stimulus generator which used the Nucleus DPS version 6.125 programming software. During stimulus presentation, measurements were made using custom-designed signal-averaging equipment. Averaged reflexes were obtained in seven out of 12 children, and the muscle contraction was visually judged to be present in nine out of the 12. No comparisons were made between the intraoperative reflexes and postoperative programming levels. The authors indicated plans to continue work on development of the technique.

Summary of literature

A review of the literature regarding measurement and usefulness of ESRTs in cochlear implant users reveals a growing interest over the past 15 years. Study after study has demonstrated that the stapedial reflex can be elicited by electrical stimulation of the auditory system through a cochlear implant in the majority of patients. Investigation has shown that electrically evoked reflexes can be measured in the same manner, and share many of the same characteristics as the acoustically elicited stapedial reflex. Studies involving experienced implant users have demonstrated predictable relationships between the reflex threshold and perceptual judgements, which fall between the most comfortable listening level and the level of loudness discomfort. For patients who display reflexes, the threshold of the response falls consistently below the level of uncomfortable loudness. It is possible that reflexes may be found in individuals who have been considered not to have responses if current levels were raised beyond the level of discomfort. This possibility has not been pursued.

Studies on reflexes measured intraoperatively on anaesthetized patients show a less robust relationship with behavioural percepts, but have been demonstrated to provide benefit as a starting point for setting maximum loudness during programming. Operating room costs and the need to consider anaesthesia effects may be the most significant deterrents to intra-operative reflex measurements.

In short, measurement of electrically evoked stapedial reflexes has been shown to be a quick, non-invasive objective procedure which can provide an excellent guideline for setting levels of maximum stimulation in all types of cochlear implants for those patients who cannot provide accurate information voluntarily. Even in experienced adult implant users, maps created using reflex measurement based maximum comfort levels have been well received, and in many cases are preferred over maps with behaviourally set upper stimulation levels.

Technique

The technique described here is one that has been used routinely at the University of Miami since 1994. ESRT measurement is attempted as part of every initial stimulation, both adult and paediatric, and is a routine procedure in all follow-up programming. Prior to measurement of reflexes, thresholds are behaviourally set by the patient. Adults and older children are asked to count the stimulus presentations. A typical up–down threshold setting procedure is used. With younger children, various conditioned response techniques are employed in the setting of minimum stimulation levels.

Once thresholds are set, adult patients, as well as children with adequate language and experience, are asked to rate increasing stimulation levels on a loudness perception scale ranging from no sound to uncomfortably loud sound. Behavioural observation techniques are used to identify signs of discomfort with very young children. After these procedures are completed, reflex measurement is attempted.

Equipment

Measurement of reflexes in cochlear implant patients requires a diagnostic immittance meter together with the implant programming system. The set-up is illustrated in Figure 4.4. It can be seen in the illustration that there is no connection between the immittance equipment and the implant programming system.

Procedures

A 'cookbook' description of the ESRT procedure used at the University of Miami is contained in the appendix. As with acoustic reflexes, measurement of ESRTs requires a normal middle ear on the probe side. In general, reflexes are measured in the ear contralateral to the implant. However, reflexes have been successfully obtained at similar stimulation levels in the implanted ear, as is the case with intraoperative reflex measures. The probe is placed into the non-implanted ear and tympanometry is performed to confirm normal middle ear function.

In the University of Miami technique, the immittance meter is set to the reflex decay mode, with a 10 second time window. This method has been found to be the most efficient. With the meter set on contralateral reflex

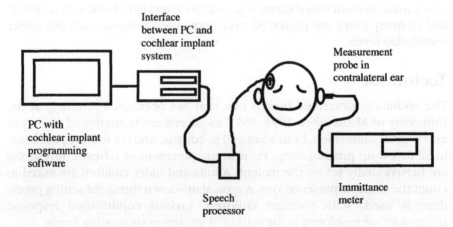

Figure 4.4. Equipment set-up for measurement of ESRTs.

measurement, no acoustic stimulation other than the probe tone is introduced to the probe ear by the immittance meter.

The patient is connected to the implant programming system via the computer interface, as is done in normal programming procedures. The stimulus that is used to elicit the reflex is always the same stimulus (same pulse width and same mode) being used to program the patient. The patient is asked to sit very still. Adults may choose to read or sleep. Children are presented with a selection of video movies that they may watch during the procedure. For children aged two or less who may not be interested in videos, they may either sleep, or be quietly amused with toys by the parent or an assistant. With the youngest children, the programming appointment may be scheduled to coincide with their usual time for sleeping.

Stimuli are presented in groups of two or three pulses; this assists in identification of the response from noise. Initial presentations are at a level that had been judged as 'loud but comfortable' in those patients who are able to provide loudness ratings. The patient is asked not to respond unless the sounds become uncomfortably loud. Children are watched carefully for any signs of discomfort. Stimulus levels are raised gradually until a response is obtained, or until the patient reports that the sound is uncomfortably loud. If at any time the patient indicates discomfort, stimulus levels will not be increased. If no reflex is obtained and uncomfortable loudness is reached on three different electrodes, testing is terminated. Once a reflex is found, stimulus levels are lowered in very fine steps until the reflex can no longer be measured (we typically use two programming units with Nucleus and MED-EL, and two fine programming steps with CLARION). Examples of reflexes obtained from both the Nucleus and CLARION devices using two different immittance systems are presented in Figure 4.5.

In the case of young children who are able to provide minimal stimulation levels through conditioned response techniques, stimulation begins at that level and is increased in large steps (10 programming units with Nucleus, five step increases with the CLARION and MED-EL) until a reflex is obtained or an indication of discomfort is noted. The levels are then dropped in fine increments until the response can no longer be measured.

In some instances a reflex is not seen at the uppermost limit of stimulation appropriate for the selected programming parameters. If this occurs, the normal procedures for increasing stimulation such as widening the stimulation mode or increasing the pulse width are employed; ESRTs have been obtained in individuals programmed in bipolar modes as wide as BP+7 (reference electrode is eight electrodes away from active electrode) using the Nucleus 22 device. Reflexes have been obtained in patients requiring wider pulse widths than the defaults in Nucleus 24, MED-EL and CLARION devices.

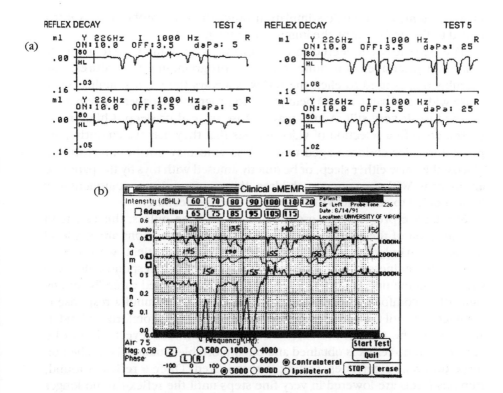

Figure 4.5. Examples of ESRTs obtained from (a) the CLARION and (b) Nucleus devices. Reflexes shown in (a) were obtained on a Grason Stadler GSI 33. Those shown in (b) were obtained on a Virtual model 310 (adapted from Figure 1 in Hodges et al., 1997).

Creating a map

With both adults and children, initial maps are made by setting maximum stimulation levels at approximately 20% below the ESRT. With the current generation of multiprogrammable speech processors, maps made at -20%, -10%, and at reflex threshold can be provided to the patient at the initial programming. Most adults find the reflex program comfortable from the start. However, those with long-term deafness, as well as young children, most often go home after initial programming using the -20% program. Adults are instructed to move to an increased maximum stimulation level programme as they feel more comfortable. Parents of young children are instructed to use the -20% program for two days and then try the -10% program. Parents are always cautioned to turn volume to the lowest setting before moving to a louder program, and to turn the sound up gradually. The same procedure is repeated until the reflex based programme is reached. If any indication of discomfort is noted, parents are instructed to return to the lower program. In most cases, even young children appear to be comfortable with maximum stimulation levels set at ESRT after several days, particularly for Nucleus device users. CLARION users are more often comfortable with upper levels set at 10% below ESRT. Limited experience gained thus far suggests that setting upper stimulation levels at reflex threshold is comfortable for MED-EL users. Volume and sensitivity are always set at the manufacturers' recommended settings.

Reflexes may be helpful in another way with the youngest cochlear implant patients. When training a child to perform a conditioned response task at the initial programming, it is often the case that the programmers are unsure that the child is even hearing the stimulus. By obtaining a reflex on even a single electrode, the programmer can be sure that the stimulation being used to condition the child is clearly audible.

Future directions

Measurement of the ESRT is a simple yet effective means of estimating upper levels of stimulation for each of the most commonly used implant systems. As with any type of objective measure, the results must be interpreted with caution. There seems to be general agreement that reflexes cannot be measured in approximately 30% of implanted patients postoperatively. In some cases, the absence can be easily explained, such as an aetiology of otosclerosis in adults. In children, especially the very young, recurrent middle-ear disorders as well as the presence of ventilation tubes can eradicate the reflex response. The reasons for lack of a reflex are more difficult to explain in other cases. Many postmeningitic individuals have apparently normal middle ears but no reflex can be obtained. This is most common among those with cochlear ossification following meningitis. The presence of a normal middle-ear response in which no reflex can be evoked can very often not be explained or related to any known factor. In older adults, it is common to find excessive flaccidity of the tympanic membrane. In such cases, the reflex is obscured by spontaneous movement of the tympanic membrane. Rhythmic movement may occur with the heartbeat or with breathing, again making it impossible to isolate the reflex from background noise using clinical immittance equipment.

In many cases such as these, it is possible that intraoperative measurement may result in a higher percentage of present reflexes. However, intraoperative reflex measurement also has limitations. As described in the literature (Van den Borne et al., 1996; Makdouhm et al., 1998), the type and amount of anaesthetic agent used, and the time period during which measurements are made can affect the threshold of the response. If the level of anaesthesia changes during the measurement procedure, the response level may be affected. In addition, if reflexes are judged visually during surgery rather than using immittance measures, the surgeon's judgement becomes a variable. Finally, if intraoperative ESRTs are to be maximally useful in postoperative programming, more research is needed into the exact relationship between the intraoperative reflex threshold and behavioural programming levels.

References

Almquist B, Harris S, Shallop JK (2000) Objective intraoperative method to record averaged electromyographic stapedius muscle reflexes in cochlear implant patients. Audiology 39: 146-52.

Battmer R, Lasig R, Lehnhardt E (1990) Electrically elicited stapedius reflex in cochlear implant patients. Ear Hear 11: 370-4.

Brown CJ, Hughes ML, Luk B, Abbas PJ, Wolaver A, Gervais J (2000) The relationship between EAP and EABR thresholds and levels used to program the Nucleus 24 speech processor: data from adults. Ear Hear 21: 151-63.

Butts SL, Hodges AV, Balkany TJ, King JE, Bricker KK, Lingvai JR (2001) Stapedial reflexes in MED-EL cochlear implant users. Presented at the CI 2001, VIth Biennial Conference on Cochlear Implants in Children, Los Angeles CA, USA.

Hodges AV, Balkany TJ, Ruth RA, Lambert PR, Dolan-Ash MS, Schloffman JJ (1997) Electrical middle ear muscle reflex: use in cochlear implant programming. Otolaryngol Head Neck Surg 117: 255-61.

Hodges AV, Balkany TJ, Ruth RA, Schloffman JJ (1996) Equal loudness balancing using electrical middle ear muscle reflexes. Presented at the International Cochlear Implant, Speech and Hearing Symposium, Melbourne, Australia.

Hodges AV, Butts SL, Dolan-Ash MS, Balkany TJ (1999) Using electrically evoked auditory reflex thresholds to fit the CLARION© cochlear implant. Ann Otol Rhinol Laryngol 108: 64-8.

Hodges AV, Butts SL, King JE, Balkany TJ (2000) Electrically elicited stapedial reflexes in Nucleus 24 cochlear implant users. Presented at CI 2000, VI International Conference on Cochlear Implants, Miami FL, USA.

Hughes ML, Brown CJ, Abbas PJ, Wolaver AA, Gervais JP (2000) Comparison of EAP thresholds to MAP levels in the Nucleus 24 cochlear implant: data from children. Ear Hear 21: 164-74.

Jerger J, Fifer R, Jenkins H, Mecklenberg D (1986) Stapedius reflex to electrical stimulation in a patient with a cochlear implant. Ann Otol Rhinol Laryngol 95: 151-7.

Jerger J, Oliver T, Chmiel R (1988) Prediction of dynamic range from stapedius reflex in cochlear implant patients. Ear Hear 9: 4-8.

Lindstrom B, Bredberg G (1997) Intraoperative electrical stimulation of the stapedius reflex in children. Am J Otol 18: 118-19.

Makhdoum MJ, Snik AF, Stollman MH, de Grood PM, Van den Broek P (1998) The influence of the concentration of volatile anaesthetics on the stapedius reflex determined intraoperatively during cochlear implantation in children. Am J Otol 19: 598-603.

Opie JM, Allum JH, Probst R (1997) Evaluation of electrically elicited stapedius reflex threshold measured through three different cochlear implant systems. Am J Otol 18 (Suppl): 107-8.

Shallop JK, Ash KR (1996) Relationships among comfort levels determined by cochlear implant patient's self programming, audiologist's programming, and electrical stapedius reflex thresholds. Ann Otol Rhinol Laryngol 166: 175–6.

Spivak LG, Chute PM (1994a) The relationship between electrical acoustic reflex thresholds and behavioral comfort levels in children and adult cochlear implant patients. Ear Hear 15: 184–92.

Spivak LG, Chute PM (1994b) Programming the cochlear implant based on electrical acoustic reflex thresholds: patient performance. Laryngoscope 104: 1225–30.

Stephan K, Welzl-Muller K, Stiglbrunner H (1988) Stapedius reflex threshold in cochlear implant patients. Audiology 27: 227–33.

Stephan K, Welzl-Muller K, Stiglbrunner H (1990) Dynamic range of the contralateral stapedius reflex in cochlear implant patients. Scand Audiol 19: 111–15.

Stephan K, Welzl-Muller K, Stiglbrunner H (1991) Acoustic reflex in patient with cochlear implants (analog stimulation). Am J Otol 12 (Suppl): 48–51.

Van den Borne B, Mens LHM, Snik AFM, Spies TH, Van den Broek P (1994) Stapedius reflex and EABR thresholds in experienced users of the Nucleus cochlear implant. Acta Otolaryngol 114: 141–3.

Van den Borne B, Snik AF, Mens LH, Brokx JP, Van den Broek P (1996) Stapedius reflex measurements during surgery for cochlear implantation in children. Am J Otol 17: 554–8.

Appendix 4.1
ESRT measurement, University of Miami protocol

Set-up

1. Connect patient to implant programming system as in programming.
2. Set programming system to the screen used for threshold and maximum loudness measurement.
3. Use parameters in the patient's map if they are currently using the device. If performing an initial stimulation, select the desired parameters.
4. Place the measurement probe of the immittance meter into the non-implanted ear. It is not necessary to use the stimulus delivery system of the immittance equipment. The stimulus will be generated by the implant programming system and will be presented through the implant to the implanted ear. The contralateral earphone should be placed to the side and will not be used.
5. When measuring reflexes on children, it is helpful to sit the child in front of a television and allow him or her to watch a video. Adults and older children may read (or sleep). It is helpful to schedule babies during their usual time for sleeping.

Procedure

1. Ensure patient is seated comfortably and understands that he or she is to sit very quietly. The adult or older child should be instructed to indicate if the sound becomes uncomfortably loud. Young children should be carefully observed during the entire procedure for signs of discomfort not related to placement of the impedance probe.
2. Obtain a seal and perform tympanometry. The patient should have a Type A (normal) tympanogram. Reflexes can be obtained in some patients with Type C (negative middle ear pressure) responses if the negative pressure is not too great.
3. Set the immittance meter to reflex decay mode. Use a short (10–15 seconds) time window. Obtain a baseline to determine if patient is sufficiently quiet; a straight line should be observed. If there is excessive noise on the trace without obvious patient movement, try repositioning the probe to obtain a tighter seal. If the patient is moving excessively, wait until he or she calms down.
4. Select the electrode for testing. It may be preferable to begin at the apical end of the array since patients often tolerate greater levels of stimulation on these electrodes.
5. If measuring from an established map, begin stimulating at or slightly below the currently set upper level (M, C, or MCL). If performing an

initial stimulation, begin at behavioural threshold and increase in small steps.

6. Present two or three stimuli through the implant. Figure 4.3 shows typical responses. After the reflex decay measurement ends, it will need to be reactivated repeatedly until all reflexes are obtained.

7. If no response is observed, raise the stimulus level (we use five current units with Nucleus, and three steps with both MED-EL and CLARION).

8. Continue to raise the current levels in small steps until a response is observed or until the patient indicates that the sound has become uncomfortable (not just loud) or an obvious level of discomfort is reached.

9. If no response is seen before reaching discomfort, repeat the same procedure on a medial electrode. If no response is obtained before discomfort on three electrodes, terminate the process.

10. If no response is obtained at stimulation limits, and there is no indication of discomfort, use the normal procedure for increasing the range of stimulation such as widening the pulse width, and repeat the procedure.

11. Once a clear response is obtained, decrease stimulation levels in very small steps until the reflex disappears. This level is used as the basis for setting upper stimulation levels.

12. Repeat this procedure for each electrode. It is not necessary to begin at threshold each time. We generally start slightly below the level obtained on the previously measured electrode.

13. Once reflex thresholds have been determined for each electrode, maps can be made. At initial stimulation we generally set the upper stimulation level at the reflex threshold for one map. Additional maps are made with increasingly larger cuts in the upper levels. Patients begin with the softest map, and increase to louder programs as they feel comfortable. Most postlingually short-term deafened adults prefer upper levels set at reflex threshold right away. Long-term deafened individuals and children need to be raised to reflex levels over a period of time. See 'Creating a map' section.

CHAPTER 5

The electrically evoked whole nerve action potential

CAROLYN J BROWN

Contents

- Introduction.
- Recording electrically evoked intracochlear potentials.
- Selection of stimulation and recording parameters.
- Basic NRT measures.
- Clinical applications.
- Future considerations.

Introduction

Acoustically evoked auditory potentials have been used routinely in audiology and otolaryngology clinics for many years. Over the course of the past two decades, cochlear implantation has moved from an experimental surgery to the treatment of choice for individuals with severe to profound sensorineural hearing loss. As cochlear implantation became more widespread, interest in recording electrically evoked auditory potentials grew; however, early attempts to record these potentials were only moderately successful. The difficulty that faced early investigators was that the evoked potential recordings that were made using electrical stimulation generally contained significant artefact contamination. Commercial instrumentation for measuring auditory evoked potentials was not designed to deal with this stimulus artefact. In addition, separating an auditory response from electrically evoked myogenic or vestibular responses was problematic. During the latter half of the 1980s and the early 1990s, techniques for recognizing and minimizing stimulus artefact became known. A number of laboratories and clinics began reporting success recording the electrically evoked auditory brainstem response (EABR) in adults and children, both via extra-cochlear promontory stimulation preoperatively and via stimulation through the implant thereafter (Van den Honert and Stypulkowski, 1986; Game et al., 1987; Miyamoto and Brown, 1987; Abbas and Brown, 1988, 1991). The relationship (or lack thereof) between these measures and speech recognition performance, as well as the relationship between EABR thresholds and the levels needed to programme the cochlear implant speech processor were defined (Shallop et al., 1991; Mason et al., 1993; Brown et al., 1994). Unfortunately, enthusiasm about using EABR clinically was never particularly high because of some very practical limitations with the technology. The most significant limitation was that the EABR, like its acoustic counterpart, is very small in amplitude and is easily affected by muscle artefact. Sedation is required to record clean, repeatable traces in an efficient manner. In addition, recording the response is time-consuming because a relatively large number of sweeps are needed to obtain a stable recording. This effectively limited the amount of data that could be recorded from an individual cochlear implant user. These limitations meant that in most of the larger cochlear implant centres, EABR recordings were made only during a very short time interval in the intraoperative period, if at all.

In 1990, a technique for recording the electrically evoked whole nerve action potential (EAP) from an intracochlear electrode in Ineraid cochlear implant users was first described (Brown et al., 1990). The speech processor of the Ineraid cochlear implant was connected to the intracochlear array via a percutaneous connector. This feature allowed an electrically isolated, differential recording amplifier to be directly connected with the electrodes in the cochlea. Brown et al. (1990) developed a technique for minimizing the electrical stimulus artefact allowing the EAP to be recorded. This was the first time that an electrically evoked auditory potential had been recorded from an intracochlear electrode in a human. The Ineraid device is no longer marketed.

As a potential clinical tool the EAP has several advantages over the EABR. First, the proximity of the recording electrode to the stimulable neural elements results in large amplitude recordings. EAP amplitudes typically range from 50 to 1,500 µV whereas EABR amplitudes rarely exceed 1.5 µV. In addition, because the recording electrode is seated in the temporal bone rather than on the scalp, muscle artefact is greatly reduced. The EAP can be recorded without sedation and does not require a particularly quiet subject. As the EAP represents neural activity from a very peripheral portion of the auditory system, it is not affected by development, attention or other cognitive factors. These factors make the EAP ideal for paediatric applications. However, children were not typically considered candidates for the Ineraid device, and so for several years the EAP was only a research tool.

In 1998 Cochlear Limited introduced the Nucleus® CI24 cochlear implant. This device was capable of two-way telemetry across the skin boundary, eliminating the need for a percutaneous connection to record the EAP. Cochlear Limited used the term Neural Response Telemetry (NRT™) for the system that was used to measure the EAP. With the introduction of NRT technology it became possible to record activity from the auditory nerve in both adults and children who received the Nucleus device. Recognizing that these recordings may have clinical significance, particularly for very young children, Advanced Bionics Corporation has recently introduced the CLARION® CII cochlear implant. This device also contains the hardware necessary to record the EAP. They refer to their system for recording the EAP with the CLARION device as Neural Response Imaging (NRI). The NRI system and software have been available in a few clinics in Europe since early 2000. They are now starting an investigational trial of the NRI system in selected centres within the USA in order to comply with FDA regulations. The Austrian company MED-EL is also currently in the process of developing a system for measuring the EAP, but as of this date no information is yet available. As such, the focus of this chapter will be on the NRT system available with the Nucleus device. This chapter will begin with an overview of how the recordings are made and then describe the range of clinical applications for this technology. The chapter concludes with some thoughts about what the future may hold.

Recording electrically evoked intracochlear potentials

The EAP is a short duration neural potential that reflects the synchronous firing of a large number of electrically stimulated auditory nerve fibres. The response itself is also referred to as the electrically evoked compound action potential (ECAP). In humans, this response consists primarily of a negative peak (often referred to as N1) with a latency of 0.2 to 0.5 ms. At high presentation levels, the initial negative peak is often followed by a less robust positive peak that is referred to as P2. The amplitude of the response should be directly proportional to the number of auditory nerve fibres responding.

In theory, the best way to record an EAP would be to stimulate a given intracochlear electrode and use the same electrode (or perhaps one that is immediately adjacent to it) to record the resulting electrically evoked neural activity. In practice, the problem is that in addition to the neural response evoked by the application of the stimulus pulse, a very large stimulus artefact will also be recorded. This stimulus artefact is often large enough to saturate the recording amplifier. Once saturated, any amplifier will require a finite amount of time to recover. Amplifier saturation is not a tremendous problem if the response that is recorded has a relatively long latency. Unfortunately, because of its very short latency, saturation of the recording amplifier and the distortion introduced by this saturation can present major problems when electrically evoked intracochlear potentials are recorded. The trick to successfully recording an EAP is to find a way to eliminate or minimize stimulus artefact in the recorded neural potential.

Several different methods have been proposed for dealing with stimulus artefact. The most direct approach is to use very short duration stimuli and a recording amplifier that has a broad frequency response, sufficient gain to record a small amplitude neural signal and the ability to come out of saturation very rapidly (within 100 to 150 μs). In addition, the response requires digitization using a very rapid sampling rate, and all of this information needs to be able to be transmitted efficiently across the skin barrier for analysis. Unfortunately, none of the currently available devices allow this approach in more than a very limited subset of subjects. Even if future cochlear implant systems include a recording amplifier with the resolution necessary to record EAP responses directly without significant artefact contamination, it is likely that there will always be a sizeable subset of patients or recording conditions where artefact contamination is still a problem. A range of different techniques for dealing with stimulus artefact contamination is described below. These techniques are reviewed here with an emphasis given to the two-pulse subtraction technique that is currently in widespread use for recording the EAP with the Nucleus device.

Alternating stimulus polarity

A common technique for minimizing stimulus artefact contamination is to alternate the polarity of the stimulus in successive presentations and to average the response that is recorded. This technique is illustrated schematically in the left panel of Figure 5.1. Use of alternating stimulus polarity when recording averaged evoked potentials will minimize both stimulus artefact and any cochlear potentials that follow the stimulus polarity. The neural response evoked by the stimulus should not reverse polarity as the stimulus polarity changes and therefore will be preserved in the average. This is a relatively simple approach and has been used successfully for many years with the ABR and the EABR.

In specific cases, alternating stimulus polarity has been shown to reduce stimulus artefact enough to allow recording of an EAP from intracochlear electrodes of human cochlear implant users (Brown et al., 1990). However the assumption underlying the success of this procedure is that the neural response is identical in response to either anodic or cathodic leading biphasic current pulses. This assumption is not always true (Van den Honert and Stypulkowski, 1987; Miller et al., 1998; Miller et al., 1999). The EAP responses measured for cathodic leading biphasic current pulses can have different latency, amplitude and threshold from similar responses measured

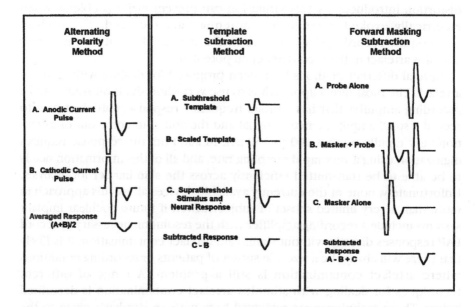

Figure 5.1. Three commonly used techniques for artefact reduction. Adapted from Figure 1 in Miller et al. (2000).

using anodic leading biphasic current pulses (Miller et al., 1999). If the latency of the neural response evoked using cathodic and anodic stimuli differs, the effect upon averaging these responses together would be to minimize the stimulus artefact, to broaden the EAP and potentially increase threshold. Whether or not the distortion of the EAP introduced by the use of alternating polarity stimuli is large enough to be clinically significant remains unclear. The system that is being developed by Advanced Bionics Corporation for recording the EAP with the CLARION implant is able to use alternation of the stimulus polarity to minimize stimulus artefact. While not currently possible with the NRT system of the Nucleus device, Cochlear Limited is currently in the process of developing a new system that will be able to do this.

Template subtraction

A second technique for reducing the effects of stimulus artefact is template subtraction (Miller et al., 1998). This is illustrated in the centre panel of Figure 5.1. Template subtraction requires collecting a response with a stimulus that is known to be below threshold. This recording should contain only stimulus artefact and serves as the template. The template is then scaled up so that the peak-to-peak amplitude of the stimulus artefact in the template matches the peak-to-peak stimulus artefact in recordings collected at levels above threshold. The EAP is extracted from stimulus artefact by subtracting the scaled template (which presumably has no neural response) from recordings made above threshold (which do contain a neural response). This very promising technique does not require alternation of stimulus polarity and can be used with a range of stimulus durations. Implementation of this procedure requires a very linear recording amplifier and a system that is able to sample the stimulus artefact accurately. It also requires a system with very low levels of ambient noise. Template subtraction will not work if the stimulus artefact saturates the recording amplifier. To date, template subtraction has been used most successfully in animal studies (Miller et al., 1999). The NRT system of the Nucleus device does not begin sampling until after the stimulus is over. This makes it difficult to implement this artefact reduction scheme in the current Nucleus system. However both Cochlear Limited and Advanced Bionics Corporation are developing software that will allow implementation of template subtraction.

Two-pulse subtraction

The artefact reduction technique that has been used most widely to record intracochlear electrical potentials is a two-pulse subtraction technique that has been described in detail in previous publications (for example Brown et al., 1990; Abbas et al., 1999). A simplified version of the subtraction technique is illustrated in the right panel of Figure 5.1 and in more detail in Figure 5.2. This technique uses a forward masking paradigm. Responses are recorded in several different stimulation conditions. First, a response is recorded using a single biphasic current pulse (a probe pulse). A second recording is then made using a two-pulse stimulus (a masker and a probe) with a very short interpulse interval (typically 500 μs or less). In the two-pulse condition, if the delay between the masker and probe is sufficiently short, neurons that fire in response to the masker will be refractory and unable to respond at the time the probe is presented. Therefore, the recording made in the two-pulse condition contains masker stimulus artefact and neural response to the masker as well as probe stimulus artefact. The assumption is that this recording will not contain a neural response to the probe pulse. A third recording is then made using a single pulse that is identical to the masker of the two-pulse sequence. The EAP is extracted by subtracting the recording made in the masker plus probe condition from the recording made in the probe alone condition. The masker alone recording is then added back to cancel any neural response to the masker that may remain. A peculiarity of the Nucleus NRT system is that in the masker alone condition, a small switching artefact is also introduced. This is shown

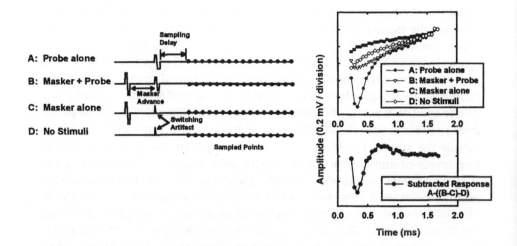

Figure 5.2. Stimulation and recording parameters associated with the Nucleus NRT system. The upper panel on the right shows the recordings made in each of four stimulation conditions (A–D). The result of the subtraction is shown in the lower right panel. Adapted from Figure 7-1 in Abbas and Brown (2000).

schematically in Figure 5.2 and requires recording of a fourth control condition that is used to subtract out the switching artefact. While this sounds convoluted and relatively complicated, it is all done automatically for the user. Figure 5.2 also illustrates how sampling is initiated after the probe pulse is presented with the Nucleus NRT system recordings and the inset shows recordings made in response to each of the individual stimulation conditions and the result of the final subtraction.

This two-pulse subtraction technique was the method originally used with Ineraid patients and later written into the Cochlear NRT software. Advanced Bionics Corporation is currently working on a version of their NRI software that will allow implementation of this subtraction method. The subtraction procedure is somewhat indirect and while there are several assumptions that underlie its use, it is still the most commonly used method of recording the EAP in both clinical and research settings today.

One drawback to the subtraction procedure is that it is not familiar or particularly intuitive to most clinicians. In addition, the amplifier used to record the EAP with the NRT system goes into saturation relatively easily. Once saturated, it tends to distort the recording in a way that is difficult to distinguish from a recording made using sub-threshold stimulation. Successful recording of the EAP using the Nucleus NRT system requires manipulation of several different parameters including the amplifier gain, the masker and probe level, the length of the interval between the masker and probe pulses, as well as the length of the delay between the offset of the probe and the initiation of sampling. In order to find the set of stimulation and recording parameters that will avoid saturation of the recording amplifier and allow the response to be recorded without significant contamination by stimulus artefact, Cochlear Limited suggests running an 'optimization series'. The purpose of the optimization series is to record systematically a set of EAP responses to fairly high-level stimuli using a combination of different gain and delay settings. The clinician then examines the set of recordings that is obtained, and the stimulation parameters that result in an optimal response morphology are selected for use with future recordings. In 1998 an 'NRT Cookbook' was published that is a fairly straightforward description aimed at the clinician, describing how to use the optimization function of the NRT software to obtain clean recordings of the EAP (Lai, 1998). At the University of Iowa we do essentially the same thing but in a slightly less formal way. For patients who use the Nucleus CI24M device, we start using a gain of 60 dB, a sampling delay of 90 µs, and a recording electrode that is located two electrodes apical to the stimulating electrode. The 'typical' settings are slightly different for patients who use the Nucleus Contour™ device. With these individuals, we start with a gain setting of 60 dB but often use recording electrodes that may be three to five electrodes away from the stimulating electrode in either direction, and a sampling delay of about 120 µs. These settings are then manipulated manually for an individual subject until a clean EAP with a clear negative peak is recorded. The settings are used to record responses for a range of stimulus levels and the whole process is repeated when the stimulating electrode is changed.

It is possible that future iterations of the hardware for recording the EAP may make this step of optimizing the response before collecting data unnecessary. In fact, it is possible that improvements in the systems used to record the EAP may make the subtraction procedure obsolete. However, as long as the subtraction procedure is used, it will still be important to understand how the choice of parameters affects the response that is recorded. That is the topic of the next section.

Selection of stimulation and recording parameters

One of the major obstacles in learning how to use the NRT system of the Nucleus device is understanding how manipulation of the different stimulation and recording parameters affects the response when the subtraction method is used to eliminate stimulus artefact. This section describes the parameters, and illustrates how manipulation of them influences the recordings. This section is specific to the Nucleus device. However future versions of the NRI software may also require the user to manipulate many of these same parameters with the CLARION device.

Stimulation mode

Monopolar stimulation is the stimulation mode that is used most widely for speech processing programs with all of the cochlear implant systems that are available today. Consequently, most clinicians and researchers are interested in the neural activity that accompanies this particular mode of stimulation. With the Nucleus device, either the ball electrode (MP1) located in the temporalis muscle or the ground electrode located on the case (MP2) can be used as the extracochlear reference. The unused reference electrode, typically MP2, is then used as a ground for the recording amplifier. It is possible with both the CLARION and the Nucleus systems, to stimulate in a bipolar mode, however, there is little information published on EAP responses recorded using bipolar stimulation.

Recording electrode position

While stimulating and recording from the same place in the cochlea would seem ideal, it is not possible with current technology. With the Nucleus NRT system, often the stimulus artefact is too large to allow for successful recording of the EAP when the recording electrode is located immediately adjacent to the stimulating electrode. This is evidenced by significant distortion or contamination of the response waveform. Figure 5.3 shows how the EAP response can be affected by the choice of the recording electrode. Data from three Nucleus cochlear implant users is shown. Two used the Nucleus CI24M device (24M-65 and 24M-66) and one was implanted with the Contour device (24R-09). The left panel of Figure 5.3 shows data collected from all three subjects using electrode 5 as the stimulating electrode. The centre and right panels show similar data obtained using electrodes 10 and 20 respectively as the stimulation electrode. The individual graphs show EAP amplitude for each subject plotted as a function of the recording electrode. In all cases, monopolar stimulation was used, and masker and probe levels were held constant. For the subject with the Contour device (24R-09) the largest amplitude responses were obtained when the recording electrode was located close to the stimulating electrode. As the recording electrode is moved away from the stimulating electrode, EAP amplitude declines. We have also observed this general pattern for subjects who use the CI24M device. For the other two subjects who use the Nucleus CI24M device the picture is a little different. For subject 24M-66, moving the recording electrode away from the stimulating electrode has very little effect on the EAP amplitude. For subject 24M-65, when electrode 10 is stimulated, the amplitude of the EAP that is recorded is much larger if the recording electrode is basal rather than apical to the

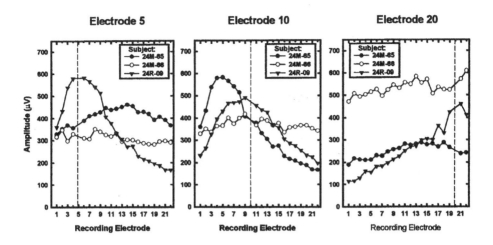

Figure 5.3. Plots showing the effect of recording electrode on EAP amplitude for three subjects. Data recorded from each of three different stimulating electrodes are shown. In each case, monopolar stimulation was used and the level of the masker and probe was held constant for all of the recordings collected from an individual subject.

stimulating electrode. For this same subject, when electrode 5 is stimulated, the maximum response amplitudes are obtained when recording electrodes are used that are located 10 electrodes away from the stimulating electrode in an apical direction.

While it is true that on average, responses obtained with the recording electrode near to the stimulating electrode tend to be larger than responses recorded from more distant sites within the cochlea, this is not true for all subjects. The 'optimization series' that is provided with the NRT software does not allow for systematic exploration of the optimal recording electrode. We generally use recording electrodes located two to three electrodes away from the stimulating electrode to record the EAP. In cases where responses are small or stimulus artefact contamination is large, we systematically vary the recording electrode position and choose the recording electrode that results in maximal response amplitudes. The data shown in Figure 5.3 suggest that varying the recording electrode in cases where less than optimal responses are observed may be beneficial.

One caveat that should be mentioned is related to the choice of recording electrode for patients who use the Nucleus Contour (CI24R) device. EAP responses recorded from electrodes 12, 14 and occasionally 16 for these subjects often appear abnormally small relative to recordings made from adjacent electrodes (for example 13, 15 and 17). This is not a problem with the device nor is it an indication that these electrodes malfunction when they are used as stimulating electrodes. The layout of the circuit for the Nucleus CI24M device and the Contour device are slightly different and it is thought that this anomaly results from additional circuit noise that is picked up when those specific electrodes (12, 14 and/or 16) are used as recording electrodes (personal communication, Cochlear Limited).

Masker and probe levels

Another variable that can have a strong effect on the EAP amplitude and response threshold is the level of the masker and probe pulses that are used. In order for the subtraction paradigm to work effectively, the masker must be equal to or higher in amplitude than the probe. Because the purpose of the masker is to put the auditory nerve fibres into a refractory state, it is often desirable for the masker to be set at a level that is near the top of the subject's dynamic range. Choosing a masker level that is equal to or exceeds the probe will ensure that any auditory neurons firing in response to the probe will have previously fired in response to the masker pulse. The masker can be left at this relatively high stimulation level and the probe level can be systematically decreased until EAP threshold is identified. This technique of fixing the masker near the top of the dynamic range and leaving it there may be optimal from a theoretical standpoint, but many clinicians hesitate to do this because they worry about potential overstimulation of the patient, particularly if that patient is a young child. The alternative is to vary the levels of the masker and probe pulses together. This may be done with the masker and probe pulses equal in intensity to each other, or with the masker varying but always 5 to 10 programming units above the probe. Figure 5.4 shows growth functions obtained from the same cochlear implant user with the three different techniques. The filled circles show the growth functions obtained using masker and probe levels that are equal but varying together. The squares and open circles show the growth functions obtained using the masker fixed at a high level and not varying while the probe level varies, and with the masker and probe levels varying together but with the masker always 10 programming units higher than the probe. These two growth functions and the resulting thresholds are virtually identical. Keeping the masker and probe pulses equal to each other and varying them together results in elevated thresholds and smaller response amplitudes. The results shown in Figure 5.4 are consistent with group results we have published previously exploring the effect of the masker and probe levels on EAP threshold and amplitude (Hughes et al., 2000b).

Typically, recording an EAP requires masker levels greater than approximately 180 programming units. For subjects with very low comfort levels, it is often difficult to record an EAP using the subtraction procedure. In situations

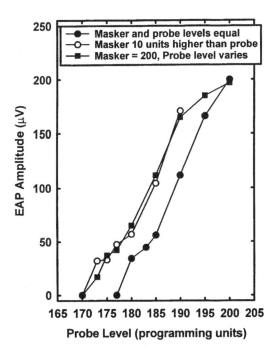

Figure 5.4. EAP growth functions recorded from a single Nucleus CI24M cochlear implant user. The function shown with filled circles was obtained by keeping the masker and probe equal in level and increasing them together. The function shown with open circles was obtained by keeping the masker 10 programming units higher than the probe at all times and varying the probe level. The function marked using filled squares was obtained by keeping the masker fixed at 200 programming units and not varying it as the probe level was varied. The same gain, recording electrode, masker advance and sampling rate was used to obtain all three growth functions.

where the patient's comfort is not an issue, for example in recordings made in the operating room, the temptation is to set the masker and/or probe levels at the maximum output levels. This is generally not effective. We have found that setting masker and probe levels too high can result in increased stimulus artefact contamination. Often decreasing the masker and/or probe amplitude slightly can resolve the artefact contamination issues and allow the EAP response to be recorded successfully.

Masker advance and sampling delay

With the most recent versions of the Nucleus NRT software, there are two different timing parameters that need to be set in order to obtain reliable NRT measures. The first is the length of the interval between the masker and the probe pulses. This is referred to as the masker advance or the interpulse interval (IPI). In order for the subtraction paradigm to work, the auditory nerve must still be in a refractory state when the probe is presented. If the interval between the masker and the probe is too long, this may not be the case. Again, however, there is a trade-off. If the probe follows the masker too closely, the amplifier may still be in saturation when the probe is presented therefore contaminating the response. Results from animal studies show that the majority of auditory nerve fibres are still in a refractory state 300 μs after the presentation of a single biphasic current pulse (Miller et al., 1999). In our work with human cochlear implant users we generally use a masker advance of 500 μs. We have found that there is a relatively small group of human subjects who have larger responses when masker advances of 300 μs rather than 500 μs are used to record the EAP. Systematically increasing the length of the masker advance results in a decrease in EAP amplitude when the subtraction method is used. This technique can be used to define the rate of recovery from the refractory state for a particular stimulation condition.

The second timing interval that needs to be specified is the delay between the offset of the probe pulse and the point at which sampling is initiated. This delay is illustrated in Figure 5.2 and is referred to as the sampling delay in the NRT software. Figure 5.5 shows a set of waveforms obtained using a range of different sampling delays. One of the unusual aspects of how the NRT system works is that once the recording amplifier is saturated, it can remain saturated for several milliseconds, effectively obscuring any response that may be present. As illustrated in Figure 5.5, if the sampling delay parameter is too short, the voltages recorded when the recording amplifier is switched in will cause saturation. If the sampling delay is too long, the response itself will be over before the sampling begins. In our experience, sampling delays less than 60 μs or longer than 150–200 μs rarely work; however, this is a parameter that needs to be manipulated for each subject and sometimes for each electrode within a subject to allow optimization of the response. We typically use sampling delays ranging from 60 to 90 μs to record EAP responses with the Nucleus CI24M device, but delays as long as 120 μs are often needed when we record EAP responses from subjects who use the Nucleus Contour device.

Amplifier gain and number of sweeps

The last set of parameters that needs to be specified is amplifier gain and the number of sweeps that are used to record an individual response. The EAP is a relatively large evoked potential; amplitudes as large as 500 μV are common and in some subjects responses have been recorded that exceed 1 mV. There are two viable options for gain with the NRT system of the Nucleus device: 40 dB and 60 dB. The default is 60 dB. Lowering the gain to 40 dB will reduce stimulus artefact and may allow for less chance of distortion of the EAP due to

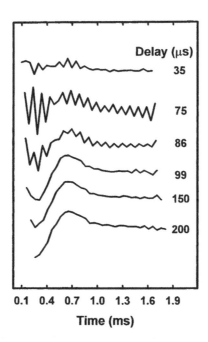

Figure 5.5. The effect of sampling delay on EAP morphology. Adapted from Figure 7 in Abbas et al. (1999).

saturation of the recording amplifier. However, the noise floor is higher when 40 dB rather than 60 dB of gain is used. We routinely use 60 dB of gain and switch to 40 dB in instances where stimulus artefact contamination is a problem. Figure 5.6 shows recordings made using single sweeps at both the 40 dB and 60 dB gain settings. Clearly the responses recorded at 40 dB are noisier and therefore more averages are needed to obtain a clean recording. The panel on the far right illustrates the effect that gain has on the EAP growth functions. Thresholds obtained using the 40 dB and 60 dB gain settings are indicated by the arrows. While not a large effect, we have found that in many subjects, the increased noise inherent in recordings obtained using the 40 dB gain setting leads to elevated thresholds and always requires more sweeps or averages to clearly define the EAP, particularly near threshold levels.

As with any evoked potential, the number of sweeps necessary to obtain a clear response is dependent on a number of factors, including both the amplitude of the response and the amount of noise in the recording. With intracochlear measures, muscle artefact is not usually an issue and the EAP is large enough that in some cases it can be recorded in a single sweep. Typically, when we use a gain setting of 60 dB we are able to record clean responses with 50 to 100 sweeps. In subjects with small amplitude responses, at stimulus levels near threshold and when 40 dB rather than

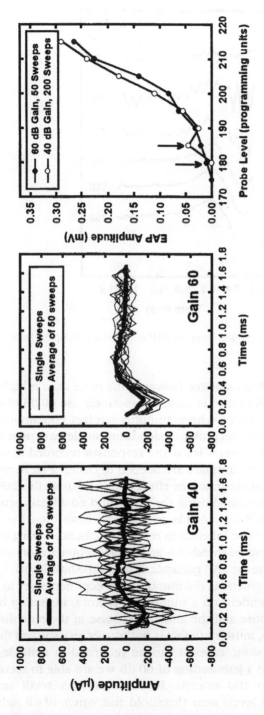

Figure 5.6. The effect of recording amplifier gain on the EAP response. The panel on the left shows ten individual recordings obtained using a gain of 40 dB. The centre panel shows ten individual recordings made from the same subject and under the same stimulation conditions but using a gain of 60 dB. The thick line in each panel shows the effect of averaging on the response. The right panel shows growth functions collected using these two different gain settings.

60 dB of gain is used, we routinely will increase the number of sweeps to between 200 and 300.

Basic NRT measures

There are three different types of measurement that can be made with the current version of the NRT software (version 2.04). These are EAP threshold, supra-threshold growth functions and refractory recovery functions. The following sections describe how these measures are obtained, issues to consider when making these measures, and their relative strengths and limitations.

EAP threshold

Perhaps the measure that has the most direct clinical application is EAP threshold. Determining EAP threshold requires the collection of a series of responses with varying probe levels. Figure 5.7 shows the screen of the NRT software used to record the EAP with the Nucleus device. The window on the left of the screen shows the individual waveforms. The stimulation level is marked in programming units. These responses are shown superimposed on each other in the lower right window and the upper right window shows the function that results when the peaks are picked and EAP amplitude is plotted relative to the probe stimulation level.

Three different methods of establishing threshold have been described. The most straightforward method is *visual detection threshold*. As the name implies, threshold is defined as the lowest level where the initial negative peak of the EAP is visible and can be replicated. This is a technique that is used widely with the auditory brainstem response (ABR). The accuracy of visual detection thresholds depends on the scale used to display the response, and on step size taken near threshold. However they have the advantage that the threshold can be identified online. In addition, determining a visual detection threshold does not require making recordings at a significant number of supra-threshold stimulation levels. This is particularly important for subjects with very restricted dynamic ranges. In Figure 5.7, the visual detection threshold is 180 clinical units.

The second method that can be used to determine EAP threshold is a method that requires collection of a more complete EAP growth function. This method has been called *linear extrapolation*. The audiologist picks the response peaks (which can be done automatically using either the Nucleus or CLARION software) for a range of probe levels. A graph of response amplitude as a function of probe level is created and linear regression techniques are used to find the equation of a line that best fits the supra-threshold data. In Figure 5.7 the linear regression line is plotted along with the data in the

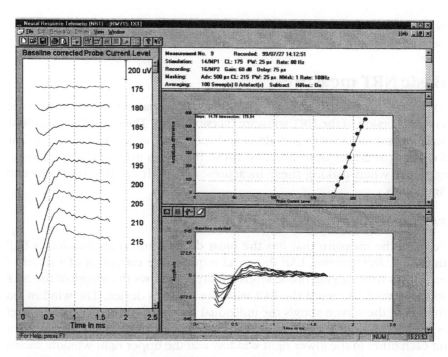

Figure 5.7. A typical EAP growth function recorded using version 2.04 of the Nucleus NRT software.

upper right window. This equation is then used to determine the stimulus level that results in a 0 μV response amplitude. The NRT software will perform this linear fit to the data automatically and the threshold that is displayed is the current level at which the linear regression intersects the x-axis. In Figure 5.7, the upper right window shows a linear extrapolation threshold of 175.54 clinical units. Linear extrapolation has the advantage that it uses more of the data collected and generally results in lower threshold levels than are found using visual detection methods. In Figure 5.7, the visual detection threshold is 180 while the threshold determined using linear extrapolation techniques is 175.54 clinical units. The disadvantage of this technique is that it assumes that the underlying form of the EAP growth function is linear. If there is saturation at high probe levels, or if there is a tail on the growth function at low stimulation level, this assumption may not be valid. Therefore rules for leaving data points out of the regression analysis must be clearly defined.

The third threshold identification technique that we have used is a technique that we refer to as *correlation threshold*. This is an offline analysis procedure that requires identification of a 'good' or 'typical' response at a supra-threshold level. This response is used as a template and cross-correlation procedures are used to compare this response with responses recorded at successively lower stimulation levels. We somewhat arbitrarily define threshold as the lowest current level that results in a correlation coefficient of 0.8. Correlation thresholds agree well with visual detection thresholds (Hughes et al., 2000b). The disadvantage of this procedure is that it is an offline analysis procedure and is not supported in the current version of the clinical NRT software. The advantage is that it can be automated, and is less dependent on the experience of the examiner than visual detection procedures.

Clearly, these three different approaches to threshold detection may yield slightly different results. The choice of which threshold detection procedure to use is dependent on many factors. For most clinical purposes, the visual detection thresholds are probably adequate. Future research, however, may show that extrapolation thresholds, which tend to be lower than either visual detection thresholds or correlation thresholds, may prove to more closely approximate map levels.

EAP growth functions

The term growth function is used to refer to a plot showing the relationship between amplitude of the EAP and probe level. Figures 5.4, 5.6 and 5.7 all show examples of EAP growth functions. EAP amplitude is dependent on the choice of masker level. If the masker is not high enough to put all of the neurons that respond to the probe into a refractory state, then EAP amplitude will be decreased (see Figure 5.4). This reasoning led us to adopt a strategy for recording EAP growth functions that required presentation of a fixed, high level masker. Probe level is varied from the point that it is equal to the masker down to threshold. Masker level is fixed at or near the maximum level tolerated by the subject. Using a fixed, high level masker ensures that the EAP amplitudes used to construct the growth function will be maximal. At the highest probe levels, where the probe level approximates the masker level, it is possible that the assumption that all of the neurons responding to the probe will also respond to the masker may not be met. The apparent saturation that occurs in EAP growth functions at high levels is artefact and results from violations of the assumptions inherent to the subtraction procedure. This saturation is illustrated in the function plotted with filled squares in Figure 5.4. The EAP amplitude versus level curve appears to roll over or flatten out at levels where the level of the probe approaches the level of the masker. This is not true saturation, it is an artefact of the subtraction technique and if these points are used in a linear regression analysis to determine EAP threshold, they can affect the results. Near threshold, if the masker level is fixed at a high level, the assumptions inherent in the subtraction procedure will very clearly be met. The disadvantage of using this technique to record the EAP growth function is that for the duration of the testing, the subject listens to a fairly intense stimulus (the fixed high level masker). Adaptation or fatigue is possible, and persistent use of high level maskers can lead to temporary increases in the subject's tinnitus. In addition, this procedure may not be as attractive for clinicians working with very young congenitally deaf children whose maximum comfort levels may not be well defined.

An alternative method of obtaining an EAP growth function uses a masker and probe whose levels are linked. This technique uses a masker that is a fixed amount above the probe. It is possible to do this automatically using the NRT software. As illustrated in Figure 5.4, EAP growth functions obtained using a fixed, high level masker and the linked masking method are essentially identical if the masker is 5 to 10 programming units higher than the probe. This is not true if the masker and probe are linked but are equal in intensity. The advantage of using the linked masker and probe levels is that a greater portion of the data collection session is spent using moderate to soft stimuli. This may be somewhat easier for subjects to tolerate rather than if a constant fixed, high level masker is used. In addition, for children, varying the masker and probe together allows the clinician to use an ascending approach and to carefully observe the child for any signs of discomfort. The disadvantage is that for subjects with small dynamic ranges, one may need to use smaller masker and probe differences in order to obtain clear suprathreshold responses.

While the primary clinical use of EAP growth functions is to determine response threshold, the slope of this function may be proportional to the number of stimulable neural elements (Smith and Simmons, 1983; Jyung et al., 1989; Hall, 1990). Many factors can influence EAP amplitude. These include the distance between the recording electrodes and the stimulable neural tissue, the impedance of the electrodes as well as the tissue within the cochlea. The slope of the EAP growth function, however, should be roughly proportioned to the number of neurons that are added for every increment in stimulation level. Steeper growth functions should be recorded from patients with more viable spiral ganglion cells.

EAP recovery functions

In addition to threshold and growth functions, the subtraction method allows us to assess the temporal response properties of the electrically stimulated auditory nerve. Specifically, it is possible to record the rate of recovery from the refractory state by holding the masker and probe levels constant and systematically manipulating the length of masker advance (the interval between offset of the masker and onset of the probe). As masker advance is increased, progressively more auditory nerve fibres will be recovered and able to respond when the probe is presented. The result is that the recording made in the two-pulse condition will contain some neural response to the probe, and this will result in a smaller amplitude response when the recording made in the masker plus probe condition is subtracted from the recording made in the probe alone condition. Figure 5.8 shows the recovery function obtained using the Nucleus NRT system. The left window shows the series of responses recorded as the masker advance was varied from 300 to 4,000 μs. Increasing the masker advance results in a systematic decrease in the response to the probe. This occurs because as the interval between the masker and probe lengthens, progressively more neurons will come out of refraction and be able to respond when the probe is presented. This results in a reduced amplitude response following subtraction. A refractory recovery function is a plot showing how EAP amplitude changes as the interval between the masker and the probe is increased. We have previously reported variability in recovery functions across subjects (Brown et al., 1990; Brown et al., 1998) and across the place of stimulation in the cochlea (Brown et al., 1996). Presumably, the faster the rate of recovery from the refractory state, the better the nerve is able to code rapid temporal information.

One limitation of the NRT system is that, when responses are recorded at relatively long IPIs, they often have no clear negative peak. It is not possible

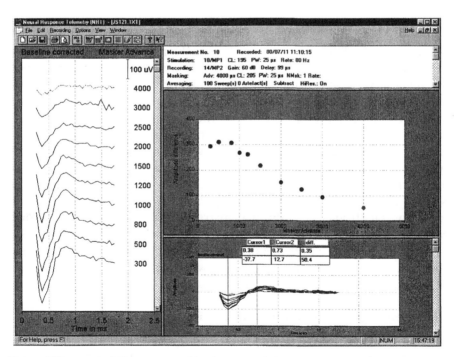

Figure 5.8. A typical EAP recovery function recorded using version 2.04 of the Nucleus NRT software.

to measure accurately the amplitude of the EAP as a function of IPI if the responses that are recorded do not have clear negative peaks. As a result, it is often not possible to fully characterize the recovery function. The basic assumption underlying the subtraction technique is that the response to the probe in the two-pulse condition where IPIs longer than 500 µs are used is a scaled-down version of the response that is recorded when the probe is presented alone. We know, by examining EAP growth functions that this is not strictly true (Miller et al., 1999). Responses recorded at low probe levels or longer IPIs can have longer response latencies and may lack a P2 peak that is present either at higher probe levels or at shorter IPIs. Miller et al. (1999) proposed an alternative technique for recording EAP recovery functions. This technique involves recording the stimulus artefact without an overlapping neural response to the probe by making a recording using two pulses and a very short IPI. A similar recording is then made using two pulses separated by a longer IPI. The recording made at the short IPI is then shifted in time and subtracted from the recording made using a longer IPI. Use of this alternative subtraction technique allows EAP recovery functions to be recorded appropriately. This technique is simple to implement offline and may be applied automatically in future version of the NRT software.

Clinical applications

Neural Response Telemetry provides a method for measuring the response of the auditory nerve to electrical stimulation. This is interesting from a theoretical point of view. Information about the auditory nerve's ability to process electrical stimuli may improve our understanding of how the auditory system processes sound and may also lead to the development of better speech coding strategies for cochlear implants. For clinicians, NRT provides the first real opportunity to record electrophysiological responses from the auditory system at the time the child first receives the cochlear implant, and at any of the routine postoperative visits. The fact that we can record this response without sedation, with minimal cooperation from the child and without recording electrodes or additional instrumentation makes this an ideal clinical tool. We still have much to learn, however, about how best to use this information to assist with the clinical management of patients with cochlear implants. The following sections review what we consider to be the most important clinical applications defined to date.

Documenting responsiveness to electrical stimulation

Perhaps the most basic clinical application for NRT is to document that the auditory nerve is able to respond to electrical stimulation. Typically, this is established in the operating room at the time of surgery. If an EAP is recorded using stimulation parameters that are typical of those used for programming, the odds are good that the child will be able to hear with the device. This may not come as a surprise for professionals working with cochlear implant patients, but such news is always reassuring for families who have had much more negative outcomes from hearing tests in the past.

In general, the time constraints in the operating room can be quite severe and can limit the amount of time available for testing. Consequently, the extent of the testing carried out in the operating room can vary tremendously from one cochlear implant centre to the next. Some centres build large data collection tables and attempt to measure the response from all 22 intra-cochlear electrodes across a range of levels. To maximize the amount of data that can be collected, very few sweeps are averaged and the stimulation and recording parameters are held constant as the recording and stimulating electrodes are systematically varied from one end of the cochlea to the other. This approach often leads to the recording of responses with missing negative peaks, but it should work well to determine which electrodes are stimulable and to gain some idea of how sensitivity changes as a function of electrode location. The accuracy of threshold determinations, however, will depend on the quality of the response recorded and the step size used. An alternative approach is to take more time to manipulate the recording and stimulation parameters (such as delay, recording electrode, gain) to obtain a response with a clear negative peak and concentrate on recording data from fewer electrodes. Both approaches work well to establish sensitivity to electrical stimulation.

Obtaining clean responses using NRT in the operating room is a reassuring sign. Those cases with no response at the time of surgery are more problematic. The challenge when this occurs is determining if this is truly a non-stimulable ear, or if there is some reason why the recording system has saturated yielding a flat recording. There are several reasons why the recordings made in the operating room may show no response in an ear that will later respond to electrical stimulation. First, the level of electrical noise in the operating room can be quite high. While NRT recordings are generally not susceptible to contamination by electrical artefact, it is possible that this may occur. Second, the tendency is to use very high stimulation and recording levels in the operating room because the patient is anaesthetized and will not have tolerance problems. Using very high stimulation levels can saturate the recording amplifier. Typically, it is not necessary to increase the stimulation levels above about 230 programming units. If we see no response initially we will often decrease the level of the masker and the probe to make sure this is not the problem. In addition, because the device has not been stimulated previously, electrode impedance can be higher for measures made in the operating room than for measures made during the postoperative period. All of these factors make recording reliable responses in the operating room more challenging. In order to minimize potential contamination by artefact or to rule out amplifier saturation, we routinely use longer sampling delays, less gain, and recording electrodes spaced further away from the stimulating electrodes to record responses in the operating room as compared with the postoperative clinic.

Based on the preceding discussion, it seems clear that the absence of a neural response in the operating room should be interpreted cautiously. We have experienced several examples of patients where no response was recorded intraoperatively (often due to excess stimulation artefact and amplifier saturation), but who then went on to stimulate and became good implant users. In many of those cases we were able to record EAP responses successfully following recovery from surgery. The patients that we are most concerned about are those with an ossified cochlea or with unusual cochlear anatomy. Unfortunately in these cases it is also possible for the electrical fields to be such that the stimulus artefact that is generated is abnormally large – a fact that can lead to increased problems with amplifier saturation. Future versions of the Nucleus NRT hardware and software may make these recordings easier to obtain.

It is also theoretically possible that the EAP may be present but the auditory nerve may be damaged enough to prevent or block conduction to the cochlear nucleus. We have never yet found a patient with an EAP who could not perceive stimulation through the device, but as more and more children with auditory neuropathy are implanted, the possibility should be considered. Caution should also be exercised in using the intraoperative measures to programme the device at initial stimulation or later. Introduction of a foreign body into the cochlea will result in development of fibrous tissue that can encapsulate the electrode array. This fibrous tissue development can change the electrical current fields in the cochlea. It is not surprising then, that the thresholds measured in the operating room can change during the postoperative period (Hughes et al., 2000a).

Obtaining a baseline and monitoring changes over time

The second clinical application for NRT is to monitor changes over time. There are two types of change that can occur. First, the device can malfunction. In some cases this malfunction is evidenced by complete lack of electrical output. In other cases, the internal receiver/stimulator may malfunction in a way that leads to inappropriate or intermittent output, or failure of only a subset of electrodes in the array. When such malfunctions occur in postlingually deafened adults, they can often be diagnosed based on patient report and/or changes in electrical impedance values. In congenitally deaf children, however, the child may not have the vocabulary or auditory experience to describe intermittencies and/or a distorted auditory percept. To complicate things further, we have had several adult patients with obviously malfunctioning electrodes based on patient report and abnormal averaged electrode voltage measures that present with normal electrode impedance values. Because failure of the internal device is a significant problem that can lead to explantation, it is very helpful to have baseline NRT measures obtained when the device was working to compare with similar measures made at a later point in time.

In addition, although it is much less common, it is possible that the internal electrode could move or extrude, resulting in increased thresholds and decreased response to electrical stimulation. Changes in neural response to electrical stimulation may also occur if a virus attacks the auditory nerve, if there is significant demyelination, or if a vestibular schwannoma begins to affect neural conduction. While all these possibilities are rare, they are examples of instances where a baseline NRT measure and/or regular monitoring of the response of the auditory nerve via NRT would be invaluable.

Much more common is the child who has been using a cochlear implant relatively successfully for a number of years and then begins to become less cooperative and to reject the device as adolescence approaches. Having an objective way of documenting that this behaviour is not due to a change in the function of the device or in his or her neural response to electrical stimulation can be reassuring to the parent and the clinician.

One of the tremendous advantages that NRT has over other auditory evoked potentials is that it is not adversely affected by muscle artefact. Prior to the introduction of NRT, if EABRs were recorded at all it was in the operating room at the time of surgery. It is possible, with NRT, to record responses from the auditory nerve at any of the routine postimplant visits. In addition, EAP thresholds have proven to be very stable for both children and adults after the first few months of stimulation. Hughes et al. (in press) report changes over time in a fairly large group of children and adults who use the Nucleus CI24M device. The EAP thresholds measured in the operating room tend to be slightly higher than those measured at the initial stimulation. The thresholds increase slightly during the first month or two after the initial stimulation, but stabilize shortly thereafter. Based on these data, it would seem reasonable to collect limited baseline information in the operating room at the time of surgery and then again on at least one visit around three months following implantation.

Assisting with the process of programming the device

The current trend in cochlear implantation is to intervene as early as possible. FDA guidelines suggest that children as young as 12 months of age may be considered for implantation. To date there have been reports of children as young as 6 months of age receiving an implant. This trend has resulted in a need for objective measures that can be used to assist with the process of fitting the speech processor of the cochlear implant. Audiologists who work with very young children are accustomed to making clinical decisions based on the results of a combination of otoacoustic emissions, immittance testing, electrophysiological thresholds and a range of different behavioural assessment procedures. A great deal of research has been published that allows the clinician to understand the relative strengths and weaknesses of all of these testing procedures. Initially, when the child is very young, more weight is given to the results of the objective testing procedures; but as the child matures, the focus shifts such that clinical decisions are more heavily weighted by the results of behavioural assessment. This process is really no different when dealing with electrical stimulation. When behavioural thresholds are either not available, unreliable or very limited, electrically evoked auditory potentials can be used to fill in the gaps. Successful use of evoked potentials (EABR or NRT) to facilitate the programming process requires, however, a pretty clear understanding of the relationship between electrically evoked thresholds and behavioural map levels.

Using NRT to predict map threshold and comfort levels

Studies have shown that the correlation between either NRT or EABR thresholds and behavioural thresholds is relatively strong if the same stimulus is used to elicit both types of responses (Abbas and Brown, 1991; Shallop et al., 1991; Brown et al., 1994). However, this is typically not the comparison of interest. The stimulus that is optimal for making EABR or NRT recordings is a continuous train of biphasic current pulses presented at a relatively slow rate, typically between 35 and 80 Hz. The stimulus used to program the speech processor is a 500 ms burst of biphasic current pulses that is repeated once every second. The frequency of the train of pulses varies depending on the programming strategy that is used. With the SPEAK programming strategy, a stimulus frequency of 250 Hz is used. With other strategies available with the Nucleus device, such as ACE™ or CIS, the stimulus can range from 250 to 2,400 Hz. In general, behavioural threshold will tend to decrease as the stimulation rate increases. This decrease in threshold observed with an increase in stimulation rate reflects the influence of temporal integration. A 500 ms burst of a 25 Hz pulse train sounds softer than a 500 ms burst of a 2,400 Hz pulse train presented at the same current level. However, temporal integration is largely a central phenomenon. While the thresholds tend to decrease as the stimulation rate is increased, similar changes in the threshold for peripherally evoked auditory potentials such as the EAP or the EABR do not occur. In fact, increasing the rate of the stimulus used to evoke the electrophysiological response will result in smaller evoked potential amplitudes and potentially also elevated thresholds.

Several investigators have reported correlations between NRT thresholds and behavioural measures of threshold (T) level and comfort (C) level for the Nucleus cochlear implant system (Brickley et al., 2000; Brown et al., 2000; Cullington, 2000; Franck and Norton, 2001). One fact common to all of these studies is that while the evoked potential thresholds and the behavioural map thresholds are correlated, there is a fairly significant amount of spread in the data. For some subjects, EAP thresholds can be recorded at levels that are close to map T levels. For other subjects, NRT thresholds more closely agree with map C levels. This fact may reflect differences in temporal integration across subjects. Subjects with relatively poor temporal integration may be expected to show minimal differences between NRT thresholds recorded at slow stimulation rates and behavioural thresholds recorded at higher stimulation rates. The opposite may be true for subjects who integrate across time more effectively. This theoretical correlation between temporal integration and the difference between EABR thresholds and map thresholds has been demonstrated for CLARION cochlear implant users (Brown et al., 1999). A technique for improving the relationship between NRT thresholds and behavioural map levels has been suggested that exploits this relationship (Brown et al., 2000; Hughes et al., 2000). This technique suggests recording EAP thresholds for each electrode across the intracochlear array and then comparing the EAP threshold recorded on one of these electrodes with behavioural measures of T and/or C level obtained for the same individual electrode using the programming stimulus. The difference between the EAP threshold and the T or C level is then used to shift the EAP threshold versus electrode function up or down by that amount in order to at least partially correct for the effects of temporal integration. This correction procedure has been described in detail in Brown et al. (2000) and when this correction is applied, the correlation between predicted T and C levels and actual 250 Hz T and C levels improves substantially.

One limitation to this procedure is that it does require that the child be able to provide a limited amount of behavioural information (for example T and/or C levels from one electrode). While application of this correction procedure may not be possible for the youngest children or for children with severe developmental delays, it may allow for more accurate programming of children who are old enough to give some indication of their dynamic range for a minimal number of electrodes, but who may not have the attention span needed to map the entire electrode array.

For children who are too young to be tested using behavioural techniques, the Hughes et al. (2000) study shows that the NRT threshold is obtained at a level where the stimulus used to program the speech processor (250 Hz pulse train for SPEAK) will rarely exceed C level. This suggests that the NRT threshold data may be used to find a level where the very young child can be conditioned to respond, and maps that are created which bracket this NRT threshold level should ensure that the auditory signal is audible for the child.

Most of the published data relating EAP thresholds to map levels has used maps programmed using the SPEAK strategy rather than the higher rate ACE or CIS strategies. Increasing the stimulus rate from the 250 Hz rate used for SPEAK to the 900 Hz used commonly for ACE results in a reduction in behavioural threshold, with a less substantial change in C levels. This effectively widens the dynamic range (Skinner et al., 2000). Figure 5.9 shows data from eight subjects who were programmed both in SPEAK and ACE (900 Hz). The functions plotted with filled symbols indicate the measured map levels. The functions plotted with open symbols show the EAP thresholds predicted using a combination of map T and C levels for electrode 10 and EAP thresholds obtained across the electrode array. The correction procedure outlined by Brown et al. (2000) should work, regardless of the frequency of the programming stimulus. Clearly for some subjects, the prediction of T and C levels based on EAP thresholds is better than for others (see for example data from subjects 24M-12 and 24M-11). In this small subject pool, increasing the stimulation rate from 250 Hz to 900 Hz does not significantly affect the accuracy of the predictions made for an individual subject. It should also be noted that increasing the stimulation rate from 250 to 900 Hz results in only minor reductions in C level for most people. The NRT thresholds recorded using an 80 Hz stimulation rate may still indicate a point where the programming stimulus is audible but comfortable even when stimulation rates higher than 250 Hz are used. More research is needed, however, to prove these assertions more fully.

Clearly there is room for improvement in our abilities to predict map levels from NRT measures and there are still a number of unanswered questions. The NRT thresholds do give us an indication of the level where the stimulus used to program the speech processor will be audible to the child. That information can be valuable because it gives the clinician a starting point for the conditioning process. We have demonstrated that at least for 250 Hz SPEAK maps, a limited amount of behavioural information (T or C level from one electrode) can be combined with the NRT measures to allow reasonable prediction of map levels. The limited data in Figure 5.9 suggest that this finding may extrapolate to the higher rate map. While maps constructed using this technique may not be perfect, they should allow us to ensure that the child who is implanted at an early age will be able to be programmed adequately until he or she is able to be programmed using more traditional techniques.

We recently used this technique to construct maps for a set of adult cochlear implant users based either primarily or entirely on NRT thresholds (Seyle and Brown, in press). We then compared speech recognition of these subjects using a map that was tuned using traditional programming procedures

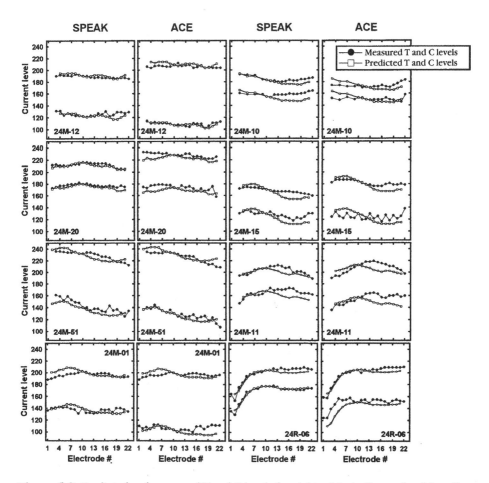

Figure 5.9. Predicted and measured T and C levels for eight subjects. For each subject, T and C levels obtained using both the 250 Hz SPEAK programming strategy and a 900 Hz ACE programming strategy are shown with filled symbols. The open symbols show predicted T and C levels made using the correction procedure describe in the text.

with maps that were based on NRT measures. Results of this study showed relatively little difference in performance on tests of word recognition with these three different maps. While the quality of sound using NRT-based maps was not perfect, the fact that they were adequate to support high levels of word recognition in adults should be reassuring to clinicians and parents of paediatric cochlear implant users. In addition, we have had cases where clinical testing suggested that a child may have an unusual map contour; for example, a range of electrodes were map levels seem particularly elevated or reduced relative to the rest of the map. Such is the case for subject 24R-06 whose data are illustrated in the two lower right panels of Figure 5.9. If these behavioural T and C levels had been obtained on a very young child, particularly one with a fairly limited attention span, the clinician may have questioned the validity of the behavioural testing. Having NRT measures that reflect this contour can be reassuring.

In the preceding discussion the results of studies describing how NRT can be used to facilitate the process of programming the speech processor of the cochlear implant have been reviewed. As with any good research project, the results raise a number of additional questions that need to be answered. First, it should be noted that when monopolar stimulation is used to program the speech processor, the maps tend to be fairly flat. As a result, studies such as those quoted above comparing NRT thresholds with map levels and pooling data across subjects with fairly large differences in behavioural threshold may result in artificially high correlation coefficients. A more rigorous way of examining these data might be to examine the within-subject correlation between electrophysiological measures and behavioural map levels.

Second, most of the data available to date were collected using subjects implanted with the Nucleus CI24 device. Recently the Contour device has been introduced, which coils more tightly around the cochlea and has smaller intracochlear electrode contacts that are spaced differently. Our experience has been that recording NRT from patients implanted with the Contour device is more difficult than for patients implanted with the CI24M device. Responses are smaller and noisier. These differences seem to be more obvious for electrodes located in the apical half of the array. This change in the internally implanted hardware, although presumably beneficial for stimulation, has seemed to have a negative effect on NRT recordings and as such, the relationship between NRT threshold and MAP levels in patients who receive the Contour device should be examined.

Third, the issue of when the NRT measures are made can be critical as well. For example, if the goal is to predict map T and C levels at the time of the initial stimulation, it may be appropriate to use NRT measures obtained in the operating room. Other clinicians may be more interested in using NRT measures recorded during the postoperative period to predict T and C levels after the map has stabilized. Both adults and children show changes over time in both NRT thresholds as well as in the behavioural levels used to construct the map (Thai-Van et al., 2001; Hughes et al., in press). In addition, both adults and children show changes in their NRT thresholds and behavioural map levels during the first few weeks after stimulation. These acute changes should be taken into account in the design of studies comparing NRT thresholds with map levels. Intraoperative measures or measures made at the initial stimulation may be more appropriately used if the goal is to predict the MAP that should be applied at the initial stimulation. If the goal is to predict MAP levels for children several months after surgery, it may be better to use NRT measures obtained during the postoperative period rather than those recorded in the operating room at the time of surgery.

Choosing a programming strategy

Finding threshold and maximum comfort levels for postlingually deafened adults is typically straightforward. However, as cochlear implant speech processors become more sophisticated, the number of signal parameters that can be manipulated has increased tremendously. As a result, it is physically impossible to have a patient (even a cooperative, postlingually deafened adult) listen to and evaluate all of the different combinations of parameters that the clinician may want to try. There is also a fairly steep learning curve during the first few weeks after the device is stimulated. The program that initially sounds the best may not yield optimal performance in the long run and, over the course of a week or two, a program that the patient is not as pleased with initially may become the best option for him. It would be ideal if some measure of neural response to electrical stimulation could be used to try to preselect stimulation parameters that would most likely result in optimal performance.

It has been suggested that NRT data may allow the preselection of optimal stimulation parameters for an individual patient, thus reducing the number of options that the patient and his or her audiologist want to explore. This would be helpful not only for adult patients but also for paediatric patients where systematically evaluating performance using a variety of different programming strategies is not possible. For example, early results with Ineraid cochlear implant users showed correlations between the rate of recovery from refraction and word recognition (Brown et al., 1990). If that is true, then one might hypothesize that patients who showed relatively rapid recovery from the refractory state may be better able to perceive rapid changes in pulse amplitude that are available with the high rate processing strategies. Patients with slower recovery functions might not be able to process these rapid changes and may do as well with a slower stimulation rate. To date, there is very little evidence that this relationship is robust enough to be adopted clinically. In general, none of the evoked potential measures show strong correlations to speech perception. However, this may change as NRT technology improves, and with increases in our understanding of how the response of the auditory nerve is related to speech perception.

Future considerations

One measure that has not been explored yet and may prove to have some utility clinically is a measure of channel interaction. The goal of multichannel cochlear implantation is to provide independent pathways of stimulation. If neural survival is very limited or if all of the surviving auditory neurons are located in one place in the cochlea, it is doubtful that placement of 22 electrodes will result in 22 separate channels of stimulation. It may, therefore, prove to be clinically useful at some point to be able to measure channel interaction.

With the current NRT software (version 2.04) channel interaction can only be measured in a very gross way by comparing plots that show stimulus amplitude plotted as a function of the recording electrode used. If there is little channel interaction, one might expect that these functions would be steeper than if there is a great deal of channel interaction (see Figure 5.3). This is a fairly time-consuming method for measuring channel interaction and may not be very sensitive.

The newest version of the NRT software (version 3.0) is currently undergoing testing at number of sites across the country. This software allows the user to choose a different electrode for the masker and the probe pulses. By comparing the response recorded with the masker and probe on the same electrode with the response recorded with the masker and probe on different electrodes, it should be possible to assess the degree to which the two channels of stimulation interact. If the electrode to which the masker is applied and the electrode to which the probe is applied stimulate the same neural population (maximum channel interaction), then EAP amplitude will be no different than the case where the masker and probe are applied to the same electrode. If, however, the masker and probe electrodes stimulate two distinct neural populations (minimal channel interaction) then no response will be recorded when the subtraction method is used. Pilot data from our laboratory suggest that this may be a reasonable way to measure channel interaction and that this measure can vary across patients. It is possible that this might be used to select a subset of electrodes to use for some of the higher rate processing schemes like CIS where channel independence is critical.

The other major difference between versions 2.04 and 3.0 of the NRT software is that with the newer software it is possible to measure NRT responses to a wider range of stimulation rates. Increasing the stimulation rate to 250 Hz results in a small but significant decrease in NRT amplitudes and a slight increase in threshold. Whether or not the use of higher stimulation rates will allow for more accurate prediction of map levels with the Nucleus device remains to be seen.

As with any new technology, the NRT/NRI systems available today will most likely pale in comparison with future technology. Changes that are currently planned for the NRT system of the Nucleus device include increasing the sampling rate and solving the amplifier saturation problems. Resolving these issues will require hardware changes and therefore will only be available once a new internal device is introduced. These changes, however, should allow EAPs to be recorded without having to use a subtraction method to extract the response from the stimulus artefact. Presumably, if artefact reduction is needed at all, users of this new generation hardware will be able to record responses using any of the artefact reduction schemes outlined at the beginning of this chapter. This new amplifier will also most likely have a lower noise floor. This should allow us to measures responses at much lower levels within the subject's dynamic range.

The NRI software available from Advanced Bionics Corporation is only now in the process of being tested for distribution. This software looks promising, and the fact that the stimulus artefact can be recorded with this system will allow implementation of the template subtraction as well as alternating polarity and the subtraction method used with the Nucleus NRT system. In addition, it is possible to measure field potentials within the cochlea, and that information may be useful for diagnosing device malfunctions. The speech processing strategies available with the CLARION device include both analogue stimulation and high rate pulsatile stimulation. How well EAP responses recorded using the NRI software correlate with behavioural measures will need to be systematically explored.

Finally, future changes in the NRT or NRI software should allow these programs to be meshed more closely with the programming software. It should be possible, for example, to record an EAP response during the programming session and to switch back and forth easily between the two modes of stimulation. Easy access to both measures simultaneously would allow better incorporation of these measures into routine clinical practice. It is hard to predict the scope or magnitude of changes in this technology that the future holds. However, the potential for clinical impact is strong and the need for this technology is clear.

Acknowledgements

The author would like to thank Michelle Hughes, Paul Abbas, Keely Seyle and Heather South for their varied and important contributions to this chapter.

References

Abbas P, Brown C (1988) Electrically evoked brainstem potentials in cochlear implant patients with multi-electrode stimulation. Hear Res 36: 153-62.

Abbas P, Brown C (1991) Electrically evoked auditory brainstem response: growth of response with current level. Hear Res 51: 123-38.

Abbas P, Brown C (2000) Electrophysiology and device telemetry. In Waltzman SB, Cohen NL (eds) Cochlear Implants. New York: Thieme, pp. 117-33.

Abbas P, Brown C, Shallop J, Firszt J, Hughes M, Hong S, Staller S (1999) Summary of results using the Nucleus CI24M implant to record the electrically evoked compound action potential. Ear Hear 20: 45-59.

Brickley G, Conway J, Craddock L (2000) Initial results of neural response telemetry recording of electrical compound action potentials from the United Kingdom. Ann Otol Rhinol Laryngol 185 (Suppl): 9-12.

Brown C, Abbas P, Borland J, Bertschy M (1996) Electrically evoked whole nerve action potentials in Ineraid cochlear implant users: responses to different stimulating electrode configurations and comparison to psychophysical responses. J Speech Hear Res 39: 453-67.

Brown C, Abbas P, Fryauf-Bertschy H, Kelsay D, Gantz B (1994) Intra-operative and post-operative electrically evoked auditory brainstem responses in Nucleus cochlear implant users: implications for the fitting process. Ear Hear 15: 168-76.

Brown C, Abbas P, Gantz B (1990) Electrically evoked whole-nerve action potentials: data from human cochlear implant users. J Acoust Soc Am 88: 1385-91.

Brown C, Abbas P, Gantz B (1998) Preliminary experience with Neural Response Telemetry in the Nucleus CI24M cochlear implant. Am J Otol 19: 320-7.

Brown C, Hughes M, Lopez S, Abbas P (1999) Relationship between EABR thresholds and levels used to program the CLARION speech processor. Ann Otol Rhinol Laryngol 108 (Suppl): 50-7.

Brown C, Hughes M, Luk B, Abbas P, Wolaver A, Gervais J (2000) The relationship between EAP and EABR thresholds and levels used to program the Nucleus 24 speech processor: data from adults. Ear Hear 21: 151-63.

Cullington H (2000) Preliminary neural response telemetry results. Br J Audiol 34: 134-40.

Franck K, Norton S (2001) The electrically evoked whole-nerve action potential: fitting application for cochlear implants. Ear Hear 22: 289-99.

Game C, Gibson W, Pauka C (1987) Electrically evoked brainstem auditory potentials. Ann Otol Rhinol Laryngol 96 (Suppl): 94-5.

Hall RD (1990) Estimation of surviving spiral ganglion cells in the deaf rat using the electrically evoked auditory brainstem response. Hear Res 45: 123-36.

Hughes M, Abbas P, Brown C, Gantz B (2000a) Using electrically evoked compound action potential thresholds to facilitate creating maps for children with the Nucleus CI24M. In: Kim C, Chang S, Lim D (eds) Updates in cochlear implantation. Adv Otorhinolaryngol 57: 260-5.

Hughes M, Brown C, Abbas P, Wolaver A, Gervais J (2000b) Comparison of EAP thresholds with map levels in the Nucleus 24 cochlear implant: data from children. Ear Hear 21: 164-74.

Hughes M, Vander Werff K, Brown C, Abbas P, Kelsay D, Teagle H, Lowder M (in press) A longitudinal study of electrode impedance, EAP and behavioural measures in Nucleus 24 cochlear implant users. Ear Hear.

Jyung RW, Miller JM, Cannon SC (1989) Evaluation of eighth nerve integrity by the electrically evoked middle latency response. Otolaryngol Head Neck Surg 101: 670-82.

Lai W (1999) An NRT Cookbook. Basel, Switzerland: Cochlear AG.

Mason S, Sheppard S, Garnham C, Lutman M, O'Donoghue G, Gibbin K (1993) Application of intra-operative recordings of electrically evoked ABRs in a paediatric cochlear implant programme. Nottingham Paediatric Cochlear Implant Group. Adv Otorhinolaryngol 48: 136-41.

Miller C, Abbas P, Brown C (2000) An improved method of reducing stimulus artefact in the electrically evoked whole-nerve potential. Ear Hear 21: 280-90.

Miller C, Abbas P, Robinson B, Rubinstein J, Matsuoka A (1999) Electrically evoked single-fiber action potentials from cat: responses to monopolar, monophasic stimulation. Hear Res 130: 197-218.

Miller C, Abbas P, Rubinstein J, Robinson B, Matsuoka A, Woodworgh G (1998) Electrically evoked compound action potentials of guinea pig and cat: responses to monopolar, monophasic stimulation. Hear Res 119: 142-54.

Miyamoto R, Brown D (1987) Electrically evoked brainstem responses in cochlear implant recipients. Otolaryngol Head Neck Surg 96: 34-8.

Seyle K, Brown C (in press) Speech perception using maps based on Neural Response Telemetry (NRT) measures. Ear Hear.

Shallop J, VanDyke L, Goin D, Mischke R (1991) Prediction of behavioural threshold and comfort values for Nucleus 22-channel implant patients from electrical auditory brain stem response test results. Ann Otol Rhinol Laryngol 100: 896-8.

Skinner M, Holden L, Holden T, Demorest M (2000) Effect of stimulation rate on cochlear implant recipients' thresholds and maximum acceptable loudness levels. J Am Acad Audiol 11: 203-13.

Smith L, Simmons F (1983) Estimating eighth nerve survival by electrical stimulation. Ann Otol Rhinol Laryngol 92: 19-23.

Thai-Van H, Chanal J, Coudert C, Veullet E, Truy E, Collet L (2001) Relationship between NRT measurements and behavioural levels in children with the Nucleus 24 cochlear implant may change over time: preliminary report. Int J Pediatr Otorhinolaryngol 58: 153-62.

Van den Honert C, Stypulkowski P (1986) Characterization of the electrically evoked auditory brainstem response (EABR) in cats and humans. Hear Res 21: 109-26.

Van den Honert C, Stypulkowski P (1987) Temporal response patterns of single auditory nerve fibers elicited by periodic electrical stimuli. Hear Res 29: 207-22.

CHAPTER 6

The electrically evoked auditory brainstem response

STEVE MASON

Contents

- Introduction.
- The EABR and related responses.
- Recording the EABR.
- Electrically evoked auditory brainstem response before implantation.
- Electrically evoked auditory brainstem response using the cochlear implant.
- Clinical applications.
- Summary.

Introduction

Electrical stimulation of the peripheral auditory nerve evokes neural activity in the ascending auditory pathway, which can be recorded using techniques similar to those employed in conventional acoustical evoked response audiometry (ERA). These electrically evoked responses represent activity from different regions of the entire auditory pathway (Miyamoto, 1986; Shallop et al., 1990; Kileny, 1991; Kim et al., 1997; Mason, 2001), and include the electrically evoked auditory brainstem response (EABR). The EABR is a valuable objective test and is employed in many cochlear implant centres, including the Nottingham Paediatric Cochlear Implant Programme (NPCIP). In recent years the EABR has played an increasing role in the management of very young children and complex patients receiving cochlear implants.

Electrically evoked responses arise from similar generator sites to those associated with acoustical stimulation (Pelizzone et al., 1989) and therefore factors such as sleep, sedation and anaesthesia affect the responses in a similar way. It is not surprising therefore that the electrically evoked compound action potential (ECAP) and EABR have received the widest development and application in the paediatric population, analogous to electrocochleography and the auditory brainstem response (ABR) in acoustical ERA (Mason, 1993). Many characteristics of the ABR that make it a practical choice for audiological use in young children also apply to the EABR.

The EABR is a valuable tool at all stages of cochlear implantation. It can be recorded in the preoperative stage using electrical stimulation presented at the promontory or round window (Kileny et al., 1994; Mason et al., 1997). This technique, in conjunction with magnetic resonance imaging (MRI), can provide valuable information regarding the presence of intact auditory neurons and the suitability of a patient for cochlear implantation. Intraoperative electrophysiological and objective measures, including the EABR, can be used to assess the function of the implant and peripheral auditory nerve pathways at the time of surgery, and to assist with initial fitting a few weeks later (Mason et al., 1995). Postoperative recordings of the EABR can also provide valuable assistance with the management of patients who present with problems of device malfunction and difficulties with tuning.

This chapter will initially examine the EABR with respect to other electrically evoked potentials. Practical application of the EABR before and after cochlear implantation will be described, plus equipment requirements, stimulus parameters and data collection methods. The role and performance of the EABR in the routine clinic and as a tool for research and development will be discussed.

The EABR and related responses

All early investigations of the brainstem response were performed using acoustical stimulation, and our knowledge of the response has been gained mainly from this modality. This knowledge has subsequently been applied to the EABR. Indeed many characteristics of the EABR, although not all, are similar to those experienced with the ABR. One of the reasons for this is the comparability of the acoustical click with the electrical biphasic pulse from the cochlear implant. Both these stimuli have a fast onset and short duration and subsequently produce a high level of synchronization of firing of auditory nerve fibres.

Historical perspectives

In 1957, Djourno and Eyries first reported on a device that could directly stimulate the cochlea, and since then many investigators have studied the electrically generated sensation of hearing. An early study of evoked potentials to electrical stimulation was reported in guinea pigs by Meikle et al. in 1977. This was followed by a report on electrical brainstem responses in humans by Starr and Brackmann in 1979. Early attempts at recording electrically evoked potentials were also targeted at the middle latency response (EMLR) rather than the EABR (Kileny et al., 1989; Shallop et al., 1990) because of the problems of stimulus artefact. The EMLR occurs beyond 10 ms, so it is not significantly affected by stimulus artefact. However, because the EMLR is not as robust as the EABR for use in the operating theatre and in young children, this led to the development of the EABR as the preferred objective tool to assist with the management of patients.

Terminology

It is common convention to introduce a capital 'E' for electrical stimulation to denote electrically evoked responses. For example, EABR for ABR, and ECAP for the CAP in electrocochleography. Individual components of the electrically evoked response are designated by a lower case 'e' to differentiate from the acoustical counterpart. So wave V becomes wave eV. This terminology will be used throughout the chapter.

Generators of the brainstem response

The first definitive description of the ABR in humans was reported by Jewett and Williston in 1971, although Sohmer and Feinmesser first recorded these neurogenic responses in 1967. Since then, the generator sites of the classic seven waves (I to VII), arising in the first 10 ms after presentation of a click stimulus, have been extensively documented (Möller, 1999). Wave I is known to be the compound action potential of the auditory nerve and is the far-field equivalent of the CAP component in electrocochleography. Wave II is thought to arise predominantly from proximal regions of the auditory nerve, and wave III from the cochlear nucleus. The superior olivary complex is considered to be the main source of wave IV, and the lateral lemniscus wave V. Waves VI and VII are thought to arise mainly from the inferior colliculus. Although these origins of the ABR are based on acoustical stimulation with a click, it is reasonable to assume that similar structures are responsible for generation of equivalent components of the EABR when evoked by a biphasic pulse stimulus.

In the acoustical ABR, there is also a clearly defined slow wave associated with wave V, and a negative component at a latency of about 10 ms. This slow negative response is often termed SN10 after Davis and Hirsh (1979), and is thought to originate in the midbrain, probably representing post-synaptic activity within the inferior colliculus (Hashimoto, 1982). These slow components are used extensively in objective estimation of hearing threshold to assist identification of a response close to threshold. Interestingly, these slow components appear to be absent when using electrical stimulation. It is suggested that the mechanics of the cochlea influence their generation since this part of the auditory system is bypassed by the electrical stimulus.

Analysis and characteristics of the EABR waveform

Latency and amplitude of the individual components of the EABR are usually measured in a similar way to the acoustical ABR. The time period from the onset of the electrical stimulus to the vertex positive peak in the waveform is described as the latency. Amplitude of individual components is recorded as the peak-to-peak amplitude from the positive peak to the following negative trough. Input/output (I/O) graphs describe the way in which the amplitude and latency of the response components change with stimulus intensity.

A comparison of the characteristics of high suprathreshold acoustical ABR and electrical EABR waveforms is shown in Figure 6.1. These are typical waveforms evoked by the click stimulus and an electrical biphasic pulse respectively. Both of these stimuli have fast rise times and produce a high level of synchronization of firing of nerve fibres in the peripheral auditory pathway. Stimulus intensity series for the ABR and EABR are shown in Figures 6.2a and 6.2b respectively.

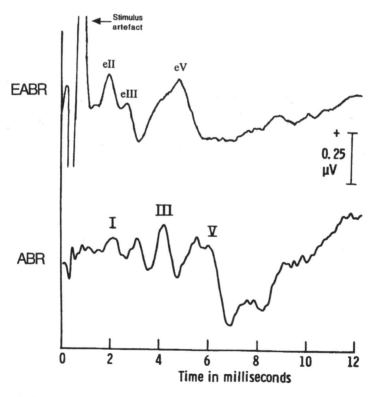

Figure 6.1. Typical response waveforms for the ABR and the EABR evoked by high suprathreshold stimulus levels.

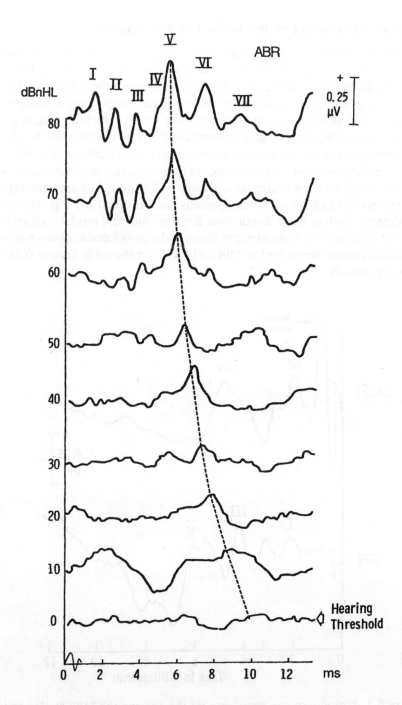

Figure 6.2a. Intensity series of waveforms for the ABR.

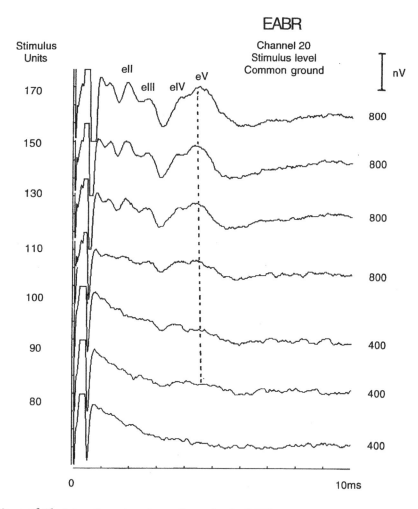

Figure 6.2b. Intensity series of waveforms for the EABR.

Although many characteristics of the EABR are similar to the ABR, there are some important differences. First, wave eI is usually obscured by the stimulus artefact and cannot be identified reliably on the EABR waveform. The latencies of the individual components of the EABR arise 1.0 to 1.5 ms earlier than the ABR (Allum et al., 1990), with wave eV occurring at about 4 to 5 ms. This is caused primarily by the electrical stimulus bypassing the transmission process of sounds through the external auditory meatus, middle ear, and along the basilar membrane (travelling wave). The EABR also behaves slightly differently with respect to changes in stimulus intensity, as shown in the input/output graphs in Figures 6.3a and 6.3b. There is only a small increase in latency with reduction in stimulus intensity. Amplitude of the response may not exhibit saturation even at relatively high stimulus levels, resulting in a steep slope on the I/O function. Close to threshold, a tailing effect (shallow slope on the I/O function) is sometimes observed. Usually wave eV is the component identified for estimation of response threshold, although in some patients waves II and III are equally dominant close to threshold. The slow components of wave V and the SN10 are remarkable by their absence in the EABR waveform.

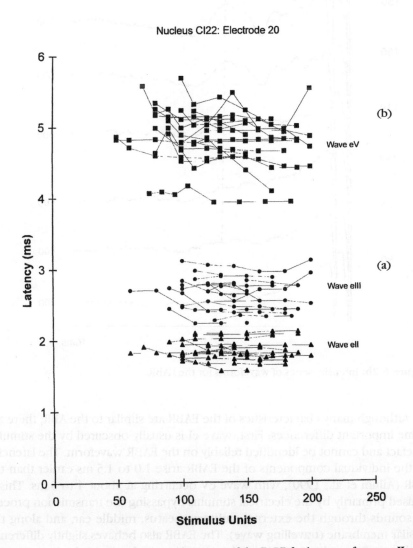

Figure 6.3a. A sample of input/output functions of the EABR for latency of waves eII, eIII and eV.

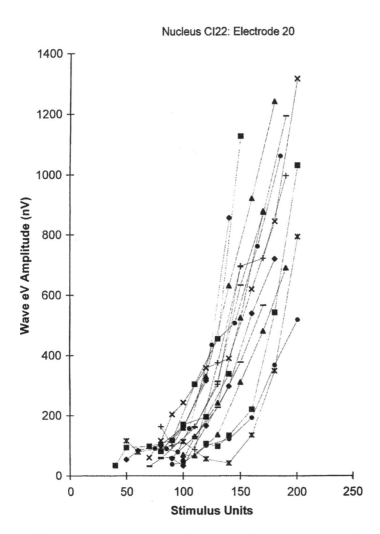

Figure 6.3b. A sample of input/output functions of the EABR for amplitude of wave eV.

The EABR waveform will be affected by brainstem maturation in a similar way to that observed with the acoustical ABR, where shorter absolute laten-cies and interpeak intervals are observed with increasing age in normally hearing neonates and young infants, most evident in the first 18 months of life. However, in cochlear implantation the picture is more complex because there is evidence that maturation of the ABR is retarded in young children with peripheral hearing loss (Walger et al., 2001). It is likely that maturation will start to recover once a child receives auditory input, such as in the case of implantation of a congenitally deaf child. A similar effect on the maturation of the auditory cortical response in children following cochlear implantation has been reported by Ponton et al. in 1999.

Short latency component (SLC)

In addition to the well-documented waves I to V of the ABR and EABR, a short latency component (SLC) can sometimes be observed on waveforms evoked by either acoustical (Mason et al., 1996) or electrical stimulation (Mason et al., 1997) as shown in Figures 6.4 and 6.5 respectively. Using a high intensity click stimulus (typically 100 dBnHL or more), the SLC is predominantly a vertex-negative component at a latency of about 3 ms. It can clearly be identified when there is no obvious response from the auditory sensory pathway, as in the case of profound hearing loss (Figure 6.4).

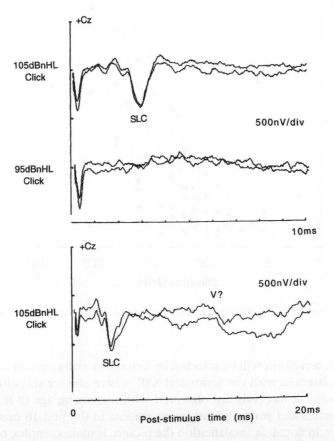

Figure 6.4. Examples of the short latency component evoked by acoustical stimulation in profound hearing loss (adapted from Figure 1 in Mason et al., 1996). The two upper traces were recorded according to a protocol for otoneurological investigation with the ABR (10 ms sweep time). The lower trace was recorded for measurement of response threshold (20 ms sweep time).

The configuration of the SLC evoked by electrical pulse stimulation is very similar to that observed with an acoustical stimulus, except that the latency of the negative component (typically 2 ms for electrical stimulation) is earlier as expected (Figure 6.5). This response has also been termed an N3 component by Kato et al. (1998). The presence of the SLC appears to be unrelated to the conventional components of the ABR because it is present both with and without a wave V or eV component. It believed to arise from stimulation of the vestibular system, with the response arising primarily from the vestibular nuclei in the brainstem.

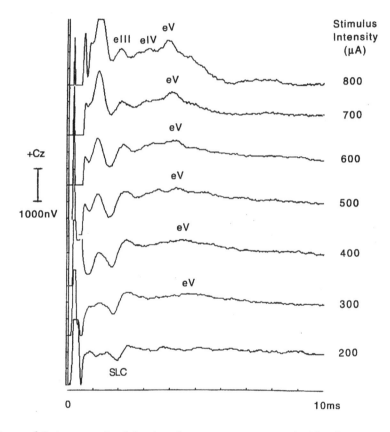

Figure 6.5. An example of the short latency component evoked by electrical stimulation during recordings of the prom-EABR.

In a study of children being assessed for cochlear implantation in the NPCIP (Mason et al., 1996) the SLC was observed in 26% of cases. Its incidence was significantly higher in congenitally deaf children (48%) compared with postmeningitic deafness (6%). Specific damage to receptors in the peripheral vestibular apparatus may be an explanation as to why the component is rarely seen in postmeningitic deafness. When the SLC was first observed in the preimplant assessments, there was concern that this may represent a retrocochlear pathology (an early component in the ABR recording with no wave V). However, we have since demonstrated that the presence of the SLC is not a contraindication for proceeding with cochlear implantation.

Compound muscle action potential (CMAP)

In addition to the neurogenic components of the EABR, a biphasic (or sometimes triphasic) compound muscle action potential (CMAP) is seen in some patients, particularly with extracochlear stimulation (Figure 6.6).

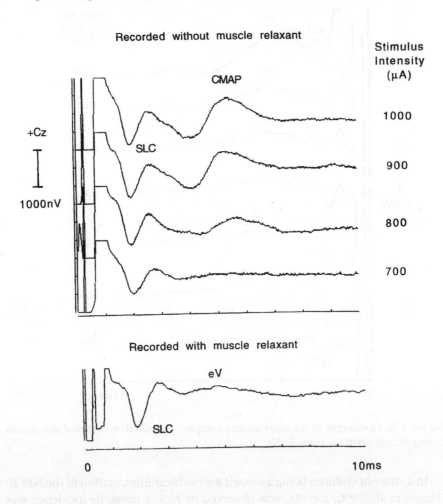

Figure 6.6. A typical compound muscle action potential evoked by electrical stimulation during an EABR recording. The lower trace shows the effect of muscle relaxant.

Excessive spread of current can cause direct stimulation of other neural pathways such as the facial nerve (Maxwell et al., 1999). The CMAP is often large when compared to the EABR and has a slightly longer latency than wave eV. Occasionally the onset of the CMAP can distort the measurement of the wave eV component. During intraoperative procedures, muscle relaxant can be administered that will abolish the CMAP, as shown in Figure 6.6.

Recording the EABR

A schematic diagram of the cochlear implant system and evoked potential equipment for performing the EABR investigation is shown in Figure 6.7. Placement of the recording electrodes on the scalp is illustrated in Figure 6.8.

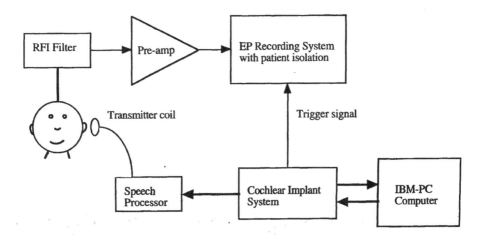

Figure 6.7. Schematic diagram of the cochlear implant system and the evoked potential equipment for EABR (Figure 6.10 in Mason, 1994).

Stimulus characteristics

The EABR is usually evoked by a biphasic electrical pulse stimulus delivered either through a single channel of an intracochlear electrode array (using the implant system); or in the case of preimplant assessment, with an extra-cochlear electrode positioned on the promontory or round window. The duration of the biphasic pulse for stimulation with the implant is typically in the range 25 to 150 μs per phase, but this usually needs to be extended to 200 or 400 μs for extracochlear stimulation. Intracochlear stimulation usually evokes an EABR that is more clearly defined than the response from an extra-cochlear stimulus.

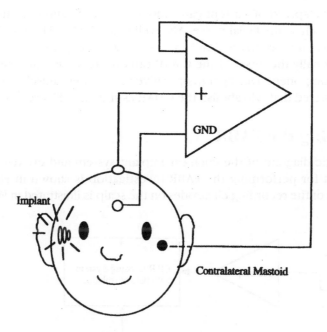

Figure 6.8. Typical placement of the scalp recording electrodes for the EABR, using the vertex and the contralateral mastoid as the active and reference sites respectively.

A train of individual pulses is required in order to record an averaged waveform, consisting of 1,000 to 2,000 sweeps. Relatively high stimulus rates can be employed (typically 85 pulses per second) because there is minimal adaptation of the individual waves of the EABR with electrical stimulation compared to the acoustical ABR (Mason et al., 1993). The adaptive mechanisms in the cochlea involved with generation of the acoustical ABR are bypassed with electrical stimulation. Fast stimulus rates enable shorter test times that are particularly valuable for young children.

Data collection

A conventional evoked potential (EP) recording system is used to acquire the data. The stimulus system and EP equipment must be accurately linked in time using a trigger pulse so that data collection is synchronized with onset of the stimulus (Figure 6.7). Most implant systems have a trigger pulse available for this purpose which can be applied to an external trigger input on the EP system. The EABR is recording from surface scalp electrodes in a similar way to the acoustical ABR, and indeed many aspects of the test parameters are similar to those employed for the acoustical ABR. However, one notable difference is the low cut-off frequency of the signal filter for the EABR. This is typically 100 Hz rather than 20 or 30 Hz because the slow components of wave V and SN10 associated with the audiological ABR (Mason, 1984) are absent in the EABR. Also a poststimulus epoch of 10 ms is sufficient to capture the whole of the EABR waveform, even with stimuli close to threshold. This is because absolute latencies are shorter than for the ABR and there is only a small shift in latency near threshold. The settings of some parameters are also influenced by the necessity to handle problems of stimulus artefact as discussed later.

Summary of typical test parameters

Electrode configuration: active = vertex (Cz).
Reference = contralateral mastoid.
Guard/common = forehead.
Amplifier sensitivity: 10 or 20 µV per display division.
Artefact rejection level: ±25 µV peak amplitude (referred to input signal).
Online signal display: ±25 µV full scale.
Filter bandwidth: 100 Hz to 3,000 Hz.
Stimulus type: biphasic electrical pulse.
Stimulus duration: in the range 25 to 400 µs per phase.
Stimulus polarity: ideally alternating onset phase to reduce stimulus artefact.
Pulse rate: 85 pps.
Sweep time: 10 ms.
Averaging sweeps: 2,000 (1,000 with high suprathreshold stimuli).
Averaged display: ±1 µV full scale (±5 µV with high suprathreshold stimuli).
Plotter output: 0.2 µV per cm (1 µV with high suprathreshold stimuli).

Handling the stimulus artefact

The main difficulty in recording good quality EABR waveforms is the stimulus artefact that arises from the radio frequency (RF) transmission signal and the electrical pulse stimulus. This can be addressed to some extent by changing the test parameters. It may be necessary to disable amplitude artefact rejection across the time period of the stimulus artefact (typically 0 to 2 ms) otherwise there will be rejection of the signal. Occasionally a low value of amplifier sensitivity (50 or 100 µV) is required, in order to avoid saturation of the signal amplifier caused by a large stimulus artefact. The RF component of the artefact can be reduced by placing a passive RF filter in line with the electrode leads (Game et al., 1990; Mason et al., 1993). The electrical component of the artefact can be reduced in the final averaged waveform by presenting a train of stimulus pulses where the onset polarity is alternately inverted during the averaging process. This is analogous to the alternately inverted polarity of the acoustical click stimulus.

Stimulus artefact must not adversely affect the performance of the signal amplifier in the EP equipment. There should be relatively quick recovery from any saturation at the onset of each sweep. Recording the signal with a very low cut-off frequency (typically 1 Hz) on the filter bandwidth can be helpful in reducing the spread of a large artefact across the EABR waveform. Some workers have employed a signal blanking circuit across the time period of the stimulus artefact (Millard et al., 1992) or have used a purpose-built preamplifier (Game et al., 1997). The electrical component of the artefact is generally larger when either the stimulating or reference electrode is extra-cochlear due to the effects of current spread.

Electrically evoked auditory brainstem response before implantation

The suitability of a cochlear implant as a means of hearing rehabilitation depends on the availability of electrically excitable auditory neurons that will subsequently result in auditory sensation and perception. The level of this neuronal survival can be investigated preoperatively using electrical stimulation to either evoke the EABR, or in adult patients to assess auditory behavioural sensation to the stimulus. Magnetic resonance imaging also has a major role to play in the preimplant assessment, but this topic is outside the scope of this chapter.

Presentation of the stimulus

The current spread from an electrical stimulus is not constrained by the mechanics of the middle ear and cochlea. It is therefore possible to apply a stimulus in the ear canal, at the promontory, or on the round window. The closer that the site of stimulation is to the cochlea, the more effective is the stimulus. Electrical stimulation with a needle electrode positioned at the round window niche or a ball electrode on the round window is considered to be more reliable and sensitive than the promontory. However, placement of the electrode at the round window requires some visualization of landmarks on the medial wall of the middle ear via a small tympanotomy or tympano-meatal flap procedure. For this reason, stimulation at the promontory has been extensively investigated, being a good compromise between a minimally invasive approach and application of an effective stimulus.

In a young child, however, the promontory or round window electrode techniques require the use of a general anaesthetic. Since evaluation of a child for implantation may already involve investigations requiring a general anaesthetic or sedation, such as ERA and imaging (CT, MRI), implementation of an additional session for electrical testing must be fully justified. One approach has been to perform the testing during surgery, immediately before implantation, while the child is already anaesthetized. We have employed this arrangement in the NPCIP as well as additional preoperative test sessions on selected children. We have also examined the possibility of combining the electrical testing with imaging under the same general anaesthetic session, but the logistics of implementing this are complicated.

Behavioural testing

An electrical stimulus can be applied to the promontory in the middle ear using a transtympanic needle electrode and many patients will experience some degree of auditory sensation. In adults the test procedure is relatively straightforward and can be performed without a general anaesthetic. However, acquiring the cooperation of older children for the test is more difficult, and in young children it becomes impossible. Alternative objective methods of testing young children are therefore required, such as recordings of the EABR.

In the early days of adult cochlear implantation, behavioural promontory testing was widely employed (Gray and Baguley, 1990). Absence of any acoustic sensation with the preoperative promontory (and round window) stimulus was taken as a contraindication for cochlear implantation (Kileny et al., 1992). However, the value of routine electrical testing as a predictor of outcome has been questioned, and many implant centres now only use the technique on selected complex adult patients. Gantz et al. (1993) reported considerable variability in the ability of preoperative behavioural promontory tests to predict audiological performance with multichannel cochlear implants.

Recording the preimplant EABR

The EABR can be evoked by an extracochlear electrical stimulus presented at the promontory or round window (Kileny et al., 1994) or even by a ball electrode placed inside the cochlea through a cochleostomy (Frohne et al., 1997). A battery-powered, custom-built stimulator is often used to present the biphasic charge-balanced pulse stimulus, since suitable commercial stimulators are not readily available. It must have constant current output so as to overcome changes in contact impedance of the stimulating electrode. Problems of stimulus artefact are exacerbated with extracochlear stimulation compared to intracochlear stimulation by the implant (Kasper et al., 1991). Some of these problems can be addressed using data collection parameters that minimize the effects of the stimulus artefact on the signal, as discussed earlier in this chapter and in Mason et al. (1997).

The EABR evoked by promontory stimulation

The characteristics of the EABR evoked by promontory stimulation (prom-EABR) are similar to those evoked by stimulation with the cochlear implant, except that the amplitude and definition of waves eII, eIII and eIV are generally reduced. Figure 6.9 shows some typical waveforms where (a) individual waves are well defined, (b) there is only a small wave eV present, and (c) the electrically evoked SLC is clearly identifiable. An intensity series for a well defined prom-EABR is shown previously in Figure 6.5. The SLC threshold in this case is clearly more sensitive than the threshold of wave eV.

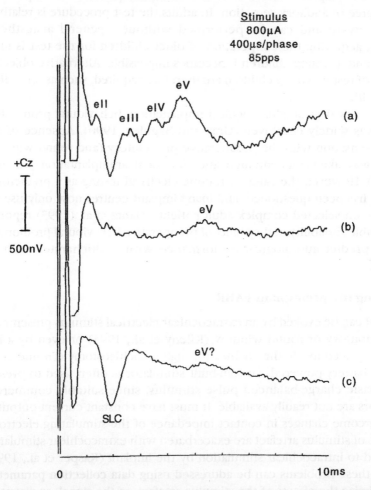

Figure 6.9. Typical EABR waveforms evoked by electrical pulse stimulation at the promontory: (a) well-defined individual components, (b) small wave eV only, (c) clearly defined SLC response (Figure 1 in Mason et al., 1997).

A compound muscle action potential (CMAP) can also be recorded on the prom-EABR waveform that can hinder the interpretation of the wave eV component. This arises from current spread resulting in stimulation of the facial nerve. However, since testing is often performed under a general anaesthetic, a muscle relaxant can be administered which inhibits the CMAP. Examples of recordings performed with and without muscle relaxant have been shown previously in Figure 6.6.

Predicting peripheral neuronal survival and outcome

There is evidence from animal studies that the amplitude input/output (I/O) function of the EABR can predict neuronal survival (Smith and Simmons, 1983). An analysis of the EABR waveforms should therefore include measurements of these characteristics (Nikolopoulos et al., 1997). In the NPCIP, the technique of recording the prom-EABR is available in the test battery. For several years the technique was used routinely during surgery (immediately before implantation) to assist with selection of the ear for implantation (Mason et al., 1997). The ear with the 'best' prom-EABR was chosen, providing there were no other factors influencing the decision, such as ossification of the cochlea or MRI imaging of the nerve bundles in the internal auditory canal. In a study of 25 children (Mason et al., 1997), the prom-EABR influenced the decision of which ear to implant in 20 cases (80%). A reliable response was recorded in 40 (80%) of the 50 ears tested. There are a number of explanations for the absence of a response: status of the auditory nerve, lack of sensitivity of the test technique, positioning of the needle electrode, and difficult recording conditions in which interpretation of the waveform was hindered by a large stimulus artefact. The incidence of absent responses is also significantly higher in children deafened after meningitis compared with congenitally deaf children (Nikolopoulos et al., 1999).

Recent experiences in the NPCIP have shown that children with no preoperative prom-EABR (wave eV) can still receive significant benefit from a cochlear implant. A study of 47 implanted children (Nikolopoulos et al., 2000) showed that children with no prom-EABR waveform (12 cases) performed as well as children with well-defined responses (35 cases). Speech perception and speech intelligibility were assessed annually up to three years after implantation using the IOWA sentence test, Connected Discourse Tracking (CDT), Categories of Auditory Performance (CAP), and Speech Intelligibility Rating (SIR). There was no statistically significant difference ($P > 0.05$) between the two groups of children using these outcome measures. Further analysis revealed that the outcome measures had not been affected by possible confounding factors (age at implantation, duration of deafness, etiology of deafness, and number of inserted electrodes). This study shows that the prognostic value of the prom-EABR is limited and absence of a prom-EABR is not, in itself, a contraindication for cochlear implantation. However, in selected cases (such as cochlear malformations, suspected cochlear nerve aplasia, narrow internal auditory canals) the presence of a prom-EABR is a positive finding in the assessment of candidates for cochlear implantation as it confirms the existence of intact auditory neurons.

In view of the results from the study by Nikolopoulos et al. (2000), the prom-EABR is no longer employed routinely to guide the selection of the ear for implantation. It is nevertheless maintained as a diagnostic tool for complex cases and provides valuable guidance regarding the decision of whether to proceed with implantation.

Assessment of central auditory pathways

The EABR will only assess the integrity of the auditory pathway up to the level of around the lateral lemniscus in the brainstem pathways, whereas other electrically evoked potentials, such as the middle latency response, and late auditory potentials will examine more central pathways. Recordings of these later potentials using promontory stimulation are possible in cooperative awake adults and older children. However, in young children the test technique requires either sedation or general anaesthesia; this adversely affects these responses and prevents reliable implementation of the technique.

An alternative approach to examine the central auditory pathways is functional MRI imaging of the auditory cortex following electrical stimulation at the promontory. Practical aspects of this technique have been reported by Obler et al. (1999) and are also under investigation in Nottingham (Alwatban et al., 2001). In the future it is hoped that this technique should enable a more comprehensive objective assessment of candidates for cochlear implantation and may provide some guidance as to the level of performance that will be achieved postoperatively.

Electrically evoked auditory brainstem response using the cochlear implant

Recordings of the EABR evoked by the cochlear implant have been investigated extensively over many years. Implementation of the technique and subsequent results are reported for implants from many of the major manufacturers:

- Advanced Bionics Corporation: CLARION® (Brown et al., 1999; Firszt et al., 1999).
- Cochlear Limited: Nucleus® (Allum et al., 1990; Shallop et al., 1991; Brown et al., 1994; Mason et al., 1994).
- MED-EL COMBI 40+ (Schmidt et al., 1998).

- MXM: Digisonic (Gallégo et al., 1998; Truy et al., 1998).
- Philips Hearing Instruments: Laura (Peeters, 1998).

Stimulus characteristics

The electrical pulse stimulus is usually delivered on a single channel of the electrode array in the scala tympani. The intensity or loudness of the stimulus perceived by the patient is dependent on electric charge, which is related to the amplitude of the current (or voltage) and the duration of the stimulus (for example pulse width). In the Nucleus Contour™ implant, stimulus intensity is expressed in arbitrary 'stimulus units' (0 to 255) that are linked to current level and stimulus duration. Other implant systems use more direct measures of current and pulse width as in the CLARION CII device (Advanced Bionics Corporation) and the COMBI 40+ (MED-EL). For an intracochlear electrode, the delivered charge is typically in the range of 10 to 200 nano-Coulombs for most implant users which is equivalent to 100 µA to 2 mA for a pulse duration of 100 µs. Some aspects of the stimulus characteristics for objective measures (such as pulse rate, pulse train) are different from those required for behavioural tuning. For this reason the programming software on many implant systems is customized for EABR measurements, including appropriate stimulus repetition rates and alternately inverted biphasic pulses for cancellation of stimulus artefact.

Investigations during surgery

Electrophysiological and objective measures at the time of implant surgery can confirm that the cochlear implant is functioning correctly and that the peripheral auditory nerve fibres are being stimulated effectively. This information provides valuable reassurance to patients, parents of young implanted children and professionals immediately after surgery. Intraoperative EABR recordings provide some of this reassurance and the results can be used in the initial fitting session to guide the selection of appropriate threshold levels of electrical stimulation. This can greatly assist progress, particularly with a child who is difficult to assess behaviourally. The EABR is also a valuable tool for monitoring either immediate re-implantation with the back-up device or later re-implantation due to implant failure (Mason et al., 2000).

Recording the EABR at the time of surgery, in addition to other objective measures, takes advantage of the patient already being anaesthetized for implant surgery. In this situation, the test conditions are good because the recording baseline will be free of movement and myogenic activity. This situation is not always easy to achieve postoperatively. Intraoperative testing is therefore popular for young children in most implant centres. The range of tests performed varies depending on the facilities and expertise available. The current NPCIP protocol includes a wide range of investigations and has always been an important part of the management of children at the time of implant surgery. The EABR is an integral part of this protocol.

The NPCIP protocol in the operating theatre

The cochlear implant programming system (for example the clinical programming system (CPS) and associated hardware for the Nucleus Contour device) and the evoked potential recording equipment are positioned in the operating theatre before the start of surgery. Attachment of scalp recording electrodes is carried out immediately after administration of the general anaesthetic and before the child is prepared for surgery. Electrode leads are colour coded for future reference as access to the scalp is not practical during the operation. After implantation of the electrode array and receiver, the transmitter coil and lead are placed in a sterile clear plastic sheath (40 mm × 1 m) and positioned over the receiver in the wound.

The EABR forms part of the following routine intraoperative protocol:

Before middle ear closure

- Back telemetry measurements of electrode impedance in common ground (CG) and monopolar 1 (MP1) modes across all 22 electrodes.
- Threshold of the electrically evoked stapedius reflex (ESR) on at least one electrode (typically electrode 11) recorded from microscopic observation of the stapedius muscle and tendon.

During wound closure

- Recordings of averaged electrode voltages (integrity testing) across all 22 electrodes in CG mode.
- Threshold of the EABR on one electrode (typically electrode 11).
- Back telemetry measurements of electrode impedance across all 22 electrodes in all available modes (CG, MP1, MP2 and MP1+2).
- Recordings of the ECAP using neural response telemetry (NRT™).

The initial back telemetry and ESR measurements are performed before the surgeon closes the middle ear. The remaining tests, which take about 30 minutes to complete, are carried out during closure of the wound and suturing of the skin flap. Implementation of this protocol therefore requires very little additional time in the operating theatre.

Assessments after implantation

The EABR can provide valuable support in the tuning and management of patients after implantation, particularly in very young children and complex cases where behavioural assessments may be difficult. Unexpected changes in threshold levels of electrical stimulation can be monitored using the EABR. However, implementation of these recordings postoperatively, particularly in a young child, is much more difficult than intraoperative testing under general anaesthesia. It may be necessary to use sedation, or even another general anaesthetic, in order to achieve sufficiently reliable test conditions. This situation will obviously restrict application of the technique to only those children in urgent need of the support of EABR measurements.

Clinical applications

Stimulation of the auditory pathway

The presence of an EABR (or ESR or ECAP) confirms that the auditory nerve fibres are receiving and reacting to electrical stimulation, and response activity is being generated in the peripheral nerve (ECAP) or brainstem pathways (EABR and ESR). Any one of these techniques is therefore an effective check of the function of the implant system and the physiological status of at least the peripheral auditory pathway. However, the EABR has been a long-standing and popular choice because it examines the higher level in the pathway. The absence of an EABR must be examined closely as it may represent a faulty electrode. Back telemetry measurements or integrity testing will help to clarify this situation.

Assistance with fitting: prediction of threshold

The EABR has been used extensively over many years to assist with fitting of the implant (Brown et al., 1994; Mason et al., 1994). The threshold of the response can guide the audiologist towards the threshold levels of electrical stimulation that are appropriate for a child. There are many reports that have shown a statistically significant relationship between the threshold of the EABR and behavioural threshold of electrical stimulation for both intraoperative and postoperative EABR (Shallop et al., 1991; Brown et al., 1994; Hodges et al., 1994; Mason et al., 1994; Gallégo et al., 1999). The accuracy of the EABR in predicting the behavioural threshold is dependent on applying appropriate correction factors. The threshold of the EABR is generally less sensitive than the behavioural threshold level (T level). The level of this offset is the result of a number of factors:

- Temporal summation effects caused by different pulse rates employed for each test (typically 31 to 85 pps for the EABR and 250 pps or higher for the T level).
- Difficulties in the identification of a small EABR close to threshold.

- In the case of intraoperative EABR, changes in the effective level of stimulation between the time of surgery and the early postoperative measurement of behavioural thresholds.

An example of this offset is described in a study of intraoperative EABR thresholds and early postoperative behavioural T levels for the Nucleus CI22M implant (Mason et al., 1994). In common ground (CG) stimulation mode, the offset between these two measures was typically around 35 units, as shown in Figure 6.10. When this offset was simply subtracted from the EABR threshold on all electrodes, it resulted in 80% of the corrected thresholds being within 30 stimulus units of the T level, and 58% within 20 units. A significant improvement in this relationship was achieved when offsets specific to a particular electrode were taken into consideration. This resulted in 98% of EABR thresholds being within 30 stimulus units of T level and 78% within 20 units.

Although many of the published reports on the application of the EABR are based on cochlear implants that have subsequently been superseded, the methods of analysis of the data are similar. However, it is vital that correction factors applied to the EABR threshold in order to predict behavioural thresholds are valid for the type of implant currently in use. For example the CI24M and the Contour device have superseded the Nucleus CI22M. As a result of

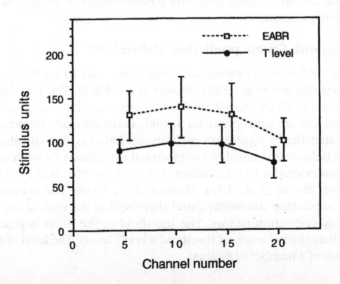

Figure 6.10. Group mean values (±1 SD) for the intraoperative EABR threshold and early behavioural T level in 24 children. The stimuli were presented via a Nucleus mini-22 electrode array in stimulus mode with a common ground (CG) reference (Figure 6.6 in Mason, 1994).

this, the default stimulus mode has changed from common ground to monopolar, where extracochlear electrodes are now used as a reference for the return current. Experience has shown that this transition in the stimulus mode significantly increases the problems of stimulus artefact on the recorded waveform due to an increase in current spread.

In addition to the EABR, the ECAP also has a role to play in the fitting process, as reported by Hughes et al. (2000). This is discussed in more detail in Chapter 5.

Dynamic range

Threshold and comfort levels for electrical stimulation define the upper and lower limits of the dynamic range. An objective prediction of the dynamic range can be derived from a combination of measurements of the EABR and the ESR. The relationship between the threshold of the ESR and comfort level of electrical stimulation is discussed in Chapter 4. In patients with a wide dynamic range, the clinical value of this prediction will be affected to a lesser extent by any inaccuracy in the EABR and ESR measurements compared to patients with a very narrow dynamic range. Additional care must therefore be exercised in applying objective predictions when the difference between the corrected thresholds of the EABR (or ECAP) and ESR is small.

Relationship of the EABR to outcome measures

A well-defined EABR waveform with a steep amplitude I/O function is thought to suggest good neuronal survival (Smith and Simmons, 1983; Hall, 1990). The presence of these characteristics of the EABR is therefore desirable but their absence is not necessarily an indicator of poor performance by the implant user. Abbas and Brown (1991) were unable to demonstrate a significant correlation between the amplitude I/O function of the implant-generated EABR and overall performance. More recently, Gallégo et al. (1998) found a statistically significant relationship between latency measures of the EABR (wave eV, and intervals eII-eV and eIII-eV) and outcome measures (phoneme recognition scores). However, many factors both peripherally and centrally influence performance with the implant, and at best the EABR alone will only account for a proportion of the variation in performance that is experienced by implant users.

Electrically evoked compound action potential (ECAP) versus EABR

A potential alternative to the EABR for intraoperative and postoperative testing is the ECAP. This can be recorded using either NRT with the Nucleus device (CI24M or Contour) or with neural response imaging (NRI) on the CLARION CII implant. Brown et al. (2000) showed that there is significant correlation between the thresholds for the EABR and ECAP (recorded using NRT). The NRT technique has the following advantages over the EABR:

- Scalp recording electrodes are not required.
- The recordings are not affected by external electrical interference.
- Children do not need to be very quiet or sedated; they can sit and play.
- Short set-up and recording times enable measurements on many electrodes.
- Particularly suited for use in the operating theatre due to lack of additional equipment required.

However, there are the following drawbacks:

- Careful selection of data collection parameters is needed for reliable recordings.
- ECAP only represents activity in the peripheral auditory system (equivalent to wave I on the ABR).
- Limited relationship between the ECAP and behavioural measures.
- Small amounts of reliable behavioural data are required for prediction of electrical threshold.

In the NPCIP, we have examined the relationship between the intraoperative recordings of the ECAP and early postoperative behavioural thresholds in young children (Mason et al., 2001). The data show an offset between the two measures that is similar to that described previously for the EABR. There is a statistically significant relationship between the two measures when intersubject variations in this offset have been taken into consideration. The offset is different for individual subjects but is similar across all the electrodes within the same subject. In other words the ECAP thresholds follow the profile of the T levels across the electrode array in any one subject.

In practice, a correction for the offset can be implemented by measuring the behavioural threshold reliably on one electrode on each individual subject at the initial tuning session (electrode 10 for example) as described by Hughes et al. (2000). The difference between this behavioural threshold and the intraoperative ECAP threshold (offset correction) is then subtracted from the absolute ECAP thresholds on all other electrodes. A high level of correlation exists once this correction has been applied, as shown in Figure 6.11 (Mason et al., 2001). This limited amount of behavioural data enables the ECAP to become a valuable predictor of behavioural threshold levels of electrical stimulation.

Recordings of the ECAP using NRT have the potential to complement or possibly replace the EABR. In straightforward cases undergoing implantation, the argument for ECAP taking priority over the EABR is strong. However in

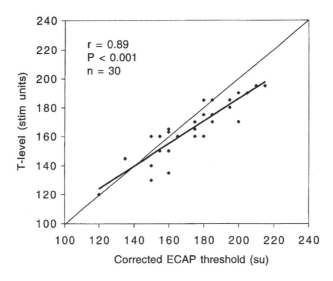

Figure 6.11. Scatterplot of offset-corrected intraoperative ECAP thresholds against early postoperative behavioural T levels. Data are presented for the Nucleus CI24M implant (electrodes 5, 15 and 20) with the offset correction derived from electrode 10. The fine diagonal line represents equal values; the bold line shows a linear regression based on these data (Figure 6 in Mason et al., 2001).

complex cases, the EABR should be retained as it provides valuable information about the integrity and functioning of brainstem pathways.

Summary

Advances in the development and application of electrophysiological and other objective measures have significantly influenced the management of patients receiving cochlear implants. The EABR has been an integral part of these electrophysiological measures over many years. The EABR will continue to be an essential diagnostic tool in implant programmes particularly as the number of implanted children with complex problems increases. There will still be a place for the EABR even when recordings of the ECAP are part of routine practice.

Acknowledgements

The author would like to acknowledge the valuable support for this work provided by the technical and scientific staff of the Evoked Potentials Clinic in the Medical Physics Department (Queen's Medical Centre, Nottingham) and the Nottingham Paediatric Cochlear Implant Programme.

References

Abbas PJ, Brown CJ (1991) Electrically evoked auditory brainstem response: growth of response with current level. Hear Res 51:123–38.

Allum JH, Shallop JK, Hotz M, Pfaltz CR (1990) Characteristics of electrically evoked 'auditory' brainstem responses elicited with the Nucleus 22-electrode intra-cochlear implant. Scand Audiol 19: 263–7.

Alwatban AZ, Ludman CN, Mason SM, O'Donoghue GM, Peters AM, Morris PG (2001) Direct electrical stimulation of the auditory system in deaf subjects: an fMRI study. Proceedings of the International Society of Magnetic Resonance Medicine, Glasgow, 2001.

Brown CJ, Abbas PJ, Fryauf-Bertschy H, Kelsay D, Gantz BJ (1994) Intra-operative and post-operative electrically evoked auditory brainstem responses in Nucleus cochlear implant users: implications for the fitting process. Ear Hear 15: 168–76.

Brown CJ, Hughes ML, Lopez SM, Abbas PJ (1999) Relationship between EABR thresholds and levels used to program the CLARION speech processor. Ann Otol Rhinol Laryngol 177 (Suppl): 50–7.

Brown CJ, Hughes ML, Luk B, Abbas PJ, Wolaver A, Gervais J (2000) The relationship between EAP and EABR thresholds and levels used to program the Nucleus CI24M speech processor. Ear Hear 21: 151–63.

Davis H, Hirsh SK (1979) A slow brainstem response for low-frequency audiometry. Audiology, 18: 445–61.

Djourno A, Eyries C (1957) Prosthese auditive par excitation electrique a distance du nerf sensoriel a l'aide d'un bobinage inclus a demeure. Presse Med 35: 14–17.

Firszt JB, Rotz LA, Chambers RD, Novak MA (1999) Electrically evoked potentials recorded in adults and pediatric CLARION implant users. Ann Otol Rhinol Laryngol 177 (Suppl): 58–63.

Frohne C, Lesinski A, Battmer RD, Lenarz T (1997) Intra-operative test of auditory nerve function. Am J Otol 18: S93–S94.

Gallégo S, Frachet B, Micheyl C, Truy E, Collet L (1998) Cochlear implant performance and electrically evoked auditory brain-stem response characteristics. Electroencephalogr Clin Neurophysiol 108: 521–5.

Gallégo S, Garnier S, Micheyl C, Truy E, Morgon A, Collet L (1999) Loudness growth function and EABR characteristics in Digisonic cochlear implantees. Acta Otolaryngol (Stockh) 119: 234–8.

Game CJA, Thomson DR, Gibson WPR (1990) Measurement of auditory brainstem responses evoked by electrical stimulation with a cochlear implant. Br J Audiol 24: 145–9.

Game CJ, Sanli H (1997) Waveforms of cochlear implant-evoked auditory brainstem responses in anesthetized young children, recorded with a new preamplifier. Ann Otol Rhinol Laryngol 106: 93–6.

Gantz BJ, Woodworth GG, Knutson JF, Abbas PJ, Tyler RS (1993) Multivariate predictors of success with cochlear implants. Adv Otorhinolaryngol 48: 153–67.

Gray RF, Baguley DM (1990) Electrical stimulation of the round window: A selection procedure for single-channel cochlear implantation. Clin Otolaryngol 15: 29–34.

Hall RD (1990) Estimation of surviving spiral ganglion cells in the deaf rat using the electrically evoked auditory brainstem response. Hear Res 45: 123–36.

Hashimoto I (1982) Auditory evoked potentials from the human midbrain: slow brain stem responses. Electroencephalogr Clin Neurophysiol 53: 652–7.

Hodges AV, Ruth RA, Lambert PR, Balkany TJ (1994) Electric auditory brain-stem responses in Nucleus multichannel cochlear implant users. Arch Otolaryngol Head Neck Surg 120: 1093-9.

Hughes ML, Brown CJ, Abbas PJ, Wolaver AA, Gervais JP (2000) Comparison of EAP thresholds with MAP levels in the Nucleus 24 cochlear implant: data from children. Ear Hear 21: 164-74.

Jewett DL, Williston JS (1971) Auditory-evoked far fields averaged from the scalp of humans. Brain 94: 681-96.

Kasper A, Pelizzone M, Montandon P (1991) Intracochlear potential distribution with intracochlear and extracochlear electrical stimulation in humans. Ann Otol Rhinol Laryngol 100: 812-16.

Kato T, Shiraishi K, Eura Y, Shibata K, Sakata T, Morizono T, Soda T (1998) A neural response with 3-ms latency evoked by loud sound in profoundly deaf patients. Audiol Neurootol 3: 253-64.

Kileny P, Kemink JL, Miller JM (1989) An intrasubject comparison of electric and acoustic middle latency responses. Am J Otol 10: 23-7.

Kileny PR (1991) Use of electrophysiologic measures in the management of children with cochlear implants: Brainstem, middle latency, and cognitive (P300) responses. Am J Otol 12: 37-42.

Kileny PR, Zwolan T, Zimmerman-Phillips S, Kemink J (1992) A comparison of round-window and transtympanic promontory electric stimulation in cochlear implant candidates. Ear Hear 13: 294-9.

Kileny PR, Zwolan TA, Zimmerman-Phillips S, Telian SA (1994) Electrically evoked auditory brain-stem response in paediatric patients with cochlear implants. Arch Otolaryngol Head Neck Surg 120: 1083-90.

Kim LS, Kang MK, Park HS, Kim SJ, Heo SD (1997) Electrically evoked auditory brainstem responses in cochlear implant patients. Adv Otorhinolaryngol 52: 92-5.

Mason SM (1984) Effects of high-pass filtering on the detection of the auditory brainstem response. Br J Audiol 18: 155-61.

Mason SM (1993) Electric Response Audiometry. In McCormick B (ed.) Paediatric Audiology 0-5 years (2nd edn). London: Whurr Publishers, pp. 187-249.

Mason SM (1994) Electrophysiological tests. In McCormick B, Archbold S, Sheppard S (eds) Cochlear Implants for Young Children. London: Whurr Publishers, pp. 103-39.

Mason SM (2001) Electrophysiological and objective tests. In McCormick B (ed.) Cochlear Implants for Young Children (2nd edition). London: Whurr Publishers (in press).

Mason SM, Sheppard S, Garnham CW, Lutman ME, O'Donoghue GM, Gibbin KP (1993) Application of intraoperative recordings of electrically evoked ABRs in a paediatric cochlear implant programme. Adv Otorhinolaryngol 48: 136-41.

Mason SM, Sheppard S, Garnham CW, Lutman ME, O'Donoghue GM, Gibbin KP (1994) Improving the relationship of intraoperative EABR threshold to T-level in young children receiving the Nucleus cochlear implant. In Hochmair-Desoyer IJ, Hochmair ES (eds) Advances in Cochlear Implants. Wein: Manz, pp. 44-9.

Mason SM, Garnham CW, Sheppard S, O'Donoghue GM, Gibbin KP (1995) An intraoperative test protocol for objective assessment of the Nucleus 22-channel cochlear implant. In Uziel AS, Mondain M (eds) Cochlear Implants in Children. Adv Otorhinolaryngol 50. Basel: Karger, pp. 38-44.

Mason SM, Garnham CW, Hudson B (1996) Electric response audiometry in young children prior to cochlear implantation: a short latency component. Ear Hear 17: 537–43.

Mason SM, O'Donoghue GM, Gibbin KP, Garnham CW, Jowett CA (1997) Perioperative electrical auditory brainstem response in candidates for pediatric cochlear implantation. Am J Otol 18: 466–71.

Mason SM, Dodd M, Gibbin KP, O'Donoghue GM (2000) Assessment of the functioning of peripheral auditory pathways after cochlear re-implantation in young children using intra-operative objective measures. Br J Audiol 34: 179–86.

Mason SM, Cope Y, Garnham J, O'Donoghue GM, Gibbin KP (2001) Intra-operative recordings of electrically evoked auditory nerve action potentials in young children by use of neural response telemetry with the Nucleus CI24M cochlear implant. Br J Audiol 35: 225–35.

Maxwell A, Mason SM, O'Donoghue GM (1999) Cochlear nerve aplasia: its importance in cochlear implantation. Am J Otol 20: 335–7.

Meikle MB, Gillette RG, Godfrey FA (1977) Comparison of electrically and acoustically evoked responses in the auditory cortex of the guinea pig: implications for a cochlear prosthesis. Trans Am Acad Opthalmol Otol 84: 183–92.

Millard RE, McAnally KI, Clark GM (1992) A gated differential amplifier for recording physiological responses to electrical stimulation. J Neurosci Methods 44: 81–4.

Miyamoto RT (1986) Electrically evoked potentials in cochlear implants. Laryngoscope 96: 178–85.

Möller AR (1999) Neural mechanisms of BAEP. Electroencephalogr Clin Neurophysiol 49 (Suppl): 27–35.

Nikolopoulos TP, Mason SM, O'Donoghue GM, Gibbin KP (1997) Electric auditory brain stem response in paediatric patients with cochlear implants. Am J Otol 18: S120–1.

Nikolopoulos TP, Mason SM, O'Donoghue GM, Gibbin KP (1999) Integrity of the auditory pathway in young children with congenital and post-meningitic deafness. Ann Otol Rhinol Laryngol 108: 327–30.

Nikolopoulos TP, Mason SM, Gibbin KP, O'Donoghue GM (2000) The prognostic value of promontory electric auditory brainstem response in pediatric cochlear implantation. Ear Hear 21: 236–41.

Obler R, Köstler H, Weber B-P, Mack KF, Becker H (1999) Safe electrical stimulation of the cochlear nerve at the promontory during functional magnetic resonance imaging. Magn Reson Med 42: 371–8.

Peeters S (1998) Objective measures with the Laura implant system. Presented at the First International Symposium and Workshop on Objective Measures in Cochlear Implantation, Nottingham UK.

Pelizzone M, Kasper K, Montandon P (1989) Electrically evoked responses in cochlear implant patients. Audiology 28: 230–8.

Ponton CW, Moore JK, Eggermont JJ (1999) Prolonged deafness limits auditory system developmental plasticity: evidence from an evoked potentials study in children with cochlear implants. Scand Audiol 28: 13–22.

Schmidt M, Klein S, Brill S (1998) Presented at the First International Symposium and Workshop on Objective Measures in Cochlear Implantation. Nottingham, UK.

Shallop JK, Beiter AL, Goin DW, Mischke RE (1990) Electrically evoked auditory brainstem response (EABR) and middle latency responses (EMLR) obtained from patients with the Nucleus multichannel cochlear implant. Ear Hear 11: 5–15.

Shallop JK, VanDyke L, Goin DW, Mischke RE (1991) Prediction of behavioural threshold and comfort values for Nucleus 22-channel implant patients from electrical auditory brain stem response test results. Ann Otol Rhinol Laryngol 100: 896-8.

Shallop J K (1997) Objective measurements and the audiological management of cochlear implant patients. In Alford BR, Jerger J, Jenkins HA (eds) Electrophysiological evaluation in otolaryngology. Adv Otorhinolaryngol 53. Basel: Karger, pp. 85-111.

Smith L, Simmons FB (1983) Estimating eighth nerve survival by electrical stimulation. Ann Otol Rhinol Laryngol 92: 19-25.

Sohmer H, Feinmesser M (1967) Cochlear action potentials recorded from the external ear in man. Ann Otol Rhinol Laryngol 76: 427-35.

Starr A, Brackmann DE (1979) Brainstem potentials evoked by electrical stimulation of the cochlea in human subjects. Ann Otol Rhinol Laryngol 88: 550-6.

Truy E, Gallego S, Chanal JM, Collet L, Morgon A (1998) Correlation between electrical auditory brainstem response and perceptual thresholds in Digisonic cochlear implant users. Laryngoscope 108: 554-9.

Walger M, Tibussek D, Foerst A, Meister H, von Wedel H (2001) Maturation of auditory brainstem responses (ABR) in children with peripheral hearing loss. Presented at the 17th Biennial Symposium of the International Evoked Response Audiometry Study Group, 22-27 July 2001, Vancouver, Canada.

CHAPTER 7

Electrically evoked middle latency and cortical auditory evoked potentials

JILL B FIRSZT, PAUL R KILENY

Contents

- Introduction.
- Recording issues with electrical stimuli.
- Middle latency response.
- Cortical auditory evoked potentials.
- Conclusion.

Introduction

The focus of electrically evoked potential studies has changed over the years as issues and concerns surrounding cochlear implantation have shifted. In the 1970s and 1980s, the unknown effects of continued use of electrical current throughout the auditory system and possible rejection of the device were primary concerns. Early researchers also were interested in whether a deaf person had an adequate supply of neurons to successfully use a cochlear implant for speech perception. Many experiments investigated the use of preimplant electrically evoked potentials to predict neural survival and postimplant performance (Walsh and Leake-Jones, 1982; Simmons and Smith, 1983; Jyung et al., 1989). For this procedure a transtympanic needle electrode is placed on the promontory, or a ball electrode in the round window niche. Electric current is then passed through the electrode as the response is recorded. In general, results with preimplant electrical recordings have been quite variable and a clear relationship between these measures and postimplant performance has not been established (Abbas, 1993).

Concerns in the 1990s related to electrical stimulation have included the decrease in the age of implantation, understanding the developmental plasticity of the nervous system in young children, estimating the number of channels needed to obtain significant levels of speech perception, and accounting for differences in speech recognition across users (NIH Consensus Statement, 1995). Because of these concerns, there has been an increase in the number of studies that incorporate electrically evoked potentials (for example, the auditory brainstem response, and middle latency response) as objective methods to investigate these questions. Due to the wide range of cochlear implant performance noted in subjects, studies of electrically evoked late latency auditory potentials generated from higher auditory centres have also increased. Since speech understanding requires both the peripheral and central systems, later potentials may serve as a window for examination of subject differences.

This chapter begins with a review of auditory middle latency responses, description of the effects of stimulus and recording variables, discussion of neural generators, and presentation of studies with both acoustic and electrical stimulation. The chapter then proceeds to the topic of late auditory evoked potentials, focusing primarily on the obligatory N1-P2 response, known to occur with the onset of a stimulus. Studies conducted to examine the central auditory system via electrically evoked potentials and possible clinical applications with cochlear implant subjects will be presented. In Chapter 8, Ponton and Don will outline in greater detail the recording methodology specific to neurophysiological responses that reflect discrimination processes, with particular attention to the mismatch negativity. Chapter 8 emphasizes research and theoretical applications of these cortical responses elicited from cochlear implant subjects. Chapters 7 and 8 both include auditory potentials generated at the level of the auditory cortex, yet with slightly different but complementary approaches to these complex neural recordings.

Recording issues with electrical stimuli

When recording electrically evoked potentials, there can be complications that interfere with response acquisition. One complication is the stimulus artefact that results from the electrical stimulus: it is large and can contaminate the neural potential of interest. This is particularly true for short latency potentials like the electrically evoked auditory brainstem response (EABR). Researchers have attempted to combat this problem with methods such as recording from the contralateral mastoid and using short biphasic pulses (Gardi, 1985; Van den Honert and Stypulkowski, 1986; Brown, 1996). Because implant systems use radio frequency (RF) signals to transmit information across the skin to the internal device, the RF signal can be picked up by the recording electrodes and can also contribute to the artefact problem. An RF filter is often needed to record successfully target responses.

Other complications that can interfere with recording early potentials involve non-auditory sensations, facial nerve stimulation and muscle artefact. Non-auditory potentials have been reported in cats (Van den Honert and Stypulkowski, 1986) but are less common in humans (Brown, 1996). In humans, facial muscle artefact has a large amplitude, grows rapidly with increased stimulus intensity, and has a latency between 5 and 10 ms (Van den Honert and Stypulkowski, 1986). In summary, the reduction of stimulus artefact is needed to improve response detectability and recognition of response contamination is important for waveform interpretation.

Middle latency response

Acoustic stimulation

The middle latency response (MLR) includes components that occur after the auditory brainstem response (ABR) but precede the late auditory evoked potentials and are known as Na, Pa, and Nb and Pb (or P1) (Picton et al., 1974). Another component within the MLR time epoch and localized over the temporal lobe is the TP41, with a latency of 45 ms (Cacace et al., 1990). The MLR waveforms tend to be larger and broader and have a relatively lower frequency spectrum than the ABR (Goldstein and Rodman, 1967; Mendel and Kupperman, 1974). Na and Pa have been studied most extensively. Across studies, Pa is the most robust component and can be recorded with stimulation rates of around 10 Hz. The latency of Na diminishes with decreases in stimulus intensity.

Earlier research with MLR components included measures of threshold, amplitude and latency to assess hearing thresholds. In adults and children, the MLR can be used, with proper precautions, to assess low- and high-frequency hearing. Responses can be recorded at levels near behavioural threshold (Picton et al., 1974; Musiek and Geurnink, 1981; Scherg and Volk, 1983; Suzuki et al., 1984; Osterhammel et al., 1985; Kraus et al., 1987). MLR research has focused on looking for generator sites and components (Scherg and von Cramon, 1986; Kraus et al., 1988; McGee et al., 1991; McGee et al., 1992), effects of maturation (Kraus et al., 1987), effects of ageing (Woods and Clayworth, 1986; Chambers and Griffiths, 1991; Chambers, 1992), and integrity of the central auditory system (Ho et al., 1987).

Important recording variables that especially affect the MLR include the presence of postauricular muscle reflex (the latency may interfere with the MLR components) and stimulus rate (slow rates are needed since cortical neurons need longer recovery periods). Employing a relatively high frequency, analogue high-pass filter setting may (by way of distortion and ringing) introduce non-existent peaks into the recording. This in turn may result in misinterpretation or an incorrect response description. Figure 7.1 (from Kileny, 1983) illustrates this point with three sets of replicated traces from the same subject, an 18-day-old male infant. Each set was recorded with different filter settings. With a bandpass filter setting of 30–100 Hz, a scalp-positive peak with a midpoint latency of 25.6 ms was obtained. When setting the low-pass filter to 1,500 Hz, the postABR scalp-positive peak had a latency of 22.8 ms. With the low-pass filter unchanged, and the high-pass filter set to 5 Hz, a broad, scalp-positive peak with a midpoint latency of 41 ms was obtained. One may conclude from this example that the positive peaks identified as Pa in the previous recordings obtained with a high-pass cut-off of 30 Hz, were the results of filter-generated oscillations triggered by the brainstem complex as suggested by Scherg (1982).

Electrode site, particularly for the non-inverting electrode, can alter the MLR. Studies by Kileny et al. (1987) and Kraus et al. (1982 and 1988) of patients with cortical lesions suggest that a response can be recorded from a midline electrode even when there is not a response from the temporoparietal area. While the MLR is affected by general anaesthesia (in particular halogenated, inhalational agents) it is possible to record the MLR in the operating room with a balanced narcotic anaesthesia such as sufentanil.

Figure 7.2 shows a sequence of acoustically evoked MLRs under sufentanil anaesthesia up to a concentration of 15 μ grams per kilogram. The main,

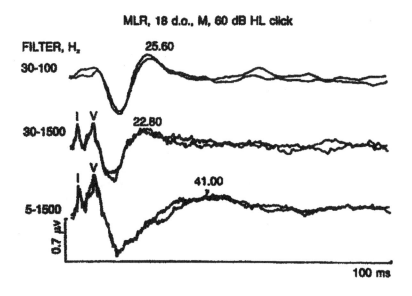

Figure 7.1. Effects of filter settings on the MLR recorded from a normally hearing 18-day-old infant. (Figure 3 in Kileny, 1983.)

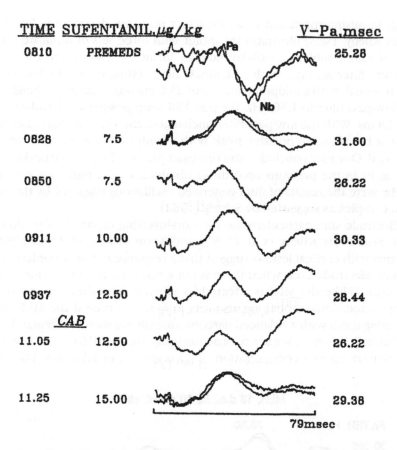

Figure 7.2. Effects of narcotic anaesthesia (sufentanil) on MLRs recorded during coronary bypass surgery. The effects include a latency prolongation and amplitude reduction of Pa, but the response persists.

systematic effect when compared to the preanaesthesia baseline (labelled 'Premeds' in the figure) is an extension of the latency of the Pa peak. Na–Pa amplitude fluctuations may also be observed, however, those were less predictable and systematic than the latency changes. In addition, because muscle relaxants were also administered along with the anaesthesia, the waveforms have a 'smoother' appearance as they are free of myogenic artefacts.

The MLR is also influenced by sleep stage: in children, Pa detectability is poor in Stage 4 sleep (Kraus et al., 1989; McGee et al., 1993). Other influencing factors include advancing age (Woods and Clayworth, 1986; Chambers, 1992) and developmental age (Jacobson, 1985; Kraus et al., 1985; Stein and Kraus, 1988). Due to maturational considerations and anaesthetic and sedative effects, MLRs are not the preferred objective measure of hearing in the very young; however, they can be useful in older children and adults. Middle latency responses can be elicited at threshold levels by both clicks and low frequency tonebursts as illustrated in Figures 7.3 and 7.4 (from Kileny and Shea, 1986). Figure 7.3 shows MLRs (top set of traces) and the 40 Hz response (a variant of the MLR obtained at a stimulus repetition rate of approximately 40 Hz) elicited by 10 dB clicks from ten normally hearing subjects (two replications from each subject). Figure 7.4 shows MLR and 40 Hz response grand averages elicited by 500 Hz tonebursts presented at 10 dB from the same subjects. Note the delay in Pa peak latency when using low frequency tonebursts.

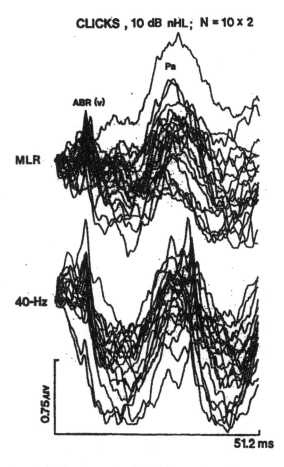

Figure 7.3. MLRs and 40 Hz responses elicited by 10 dB clicks from 10 normally hearing subjects. (Figure 2 in Kileny and Shea, 1986.)

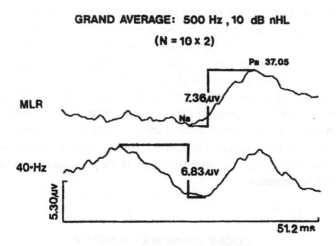

Figure 7.4. MLR and 40 Hz grand averages elicited by 10 dB 500 Hz tonebursts from 10 normally hearing subjects. (Figure 5 in Kileny and Shea, 1986.)

Middle latency response neural generators

The generators of the MLR involve a number of structures both central to the inferior colliculus and outside the primary auditory pathway. Those structures include the primary and non-primary thalamocortical pathways, and the mesencephalic reticular formation which is the midbrain arousal system that modulates attention and sleep (Buchwald et al., 1981; Kraus et al., 1988; Littman et al., 1992). Pa appears to originate from the temporal lobe region, based on data from dipole source analyses (Scherg et al., 1990) and patients with cortical lesions (Özdamar and Kraus, 1983; Scherg and von Cramon, 1986; Kileny et al., 1987). Wave Na is thought to originate from both cortical and subcortical regions, including activity from the inferior colliculus (McGee et al., 1991).

Electrical stimulation

The electrically evoked middle latency response (EMLR) has been suggested as a tool to assess the mechanisms that underlie auditory function in cochlear implant users. Recordings in animals and humans indicate that it is reliable and that waveforms are similar to the acoustic MLR (Gardi, 1985; Miyamoto, 1986; Burton et al., 1989; Kileny et al., 1989; Firszt et al., 1999). Figure 7.5 displays EMLRs recorded from one subject on an apical (electrode 1), medial (electrode 4), and basal (electrode 7) intracochlear electrode of the CLARION® cochlear implant system. A negative trough, Na, followed by a positive peak, Pa, is identified for each waveform. Response morphology is

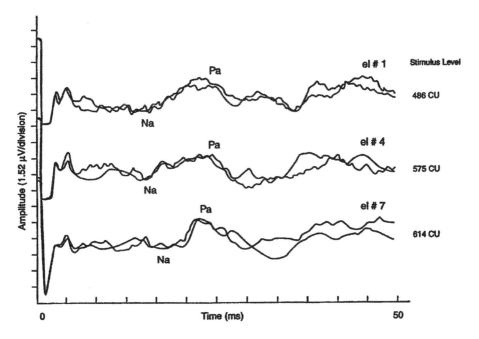

Figure 7.5. EMLR waveforms recorded from a CLARION cochlear implant user with stimulation of an apical (1), mid (4), and basal (7) electrode. Stimulus levels used to elicit the Na and Pa responses were at the upper portion of the dynamic range (adapted from Firszt, 1998).

similar across electrodes when stimulated at levels in the upper portion of the subject's electrical dynamic range. In a study by Firszt (1998), average latencies across electrodes for 11 subjects were 15.41 and 26.37 ms for Na and Pa, respectively. In this study Na–Pa amplitudes, determined between the negative Na trough and the positive peak of Pa, were 2.52 μV when averaged across electrodes for all subjects.

The EMLR is an attractive alternative to shorter latency potentials because of its longer latency (positive peak at 27 to 37 ms), making it less likely to be contaminated by the stimulus artefact that occurs early in the response. One disadvantage of the *acoustic* MLR is that it is susceptible to the influence of anaesthetics. EMLR thresholds have been obtained, however, with the use of anaesthetics (for example, nitrous oxide and narcotic anaesthetics) and without compromising the replicability of the waveforms (Kileny et al., 1989).

There has been good correspondence noted between EMLR thresholds and behavioural thresholds through the implanted electrode array (Gardi, 1985; Miyamoto, 1986; Firszt, 1998), and through transtympanic electrodes

(Kileny and Kemink, 1987). A comparison between EABR and EMLR thresholds obtained within the same subject has shown that EMLR thresholds were lower than the EABR thresholds and were closer to behavioural estimates (Gardi, 1985; Shallop et al., 1990). The latency of component Pa for electrical stimulation is consistently shorter than that for acoustic stimulation (Miyamoto, 1986; Kileny et al., 1989; Firszt et al., 2002b). The electrical Pa is larger in amplitude and narrower than its acoustic counterpart. The increased sharpness in the response is most likely due to the greater neural synchrony with electrical stimulation. Pa amplitude decreases progressively as stimulus intensity is reduced. Figure 7.6 displays the Na–Pa complex for a

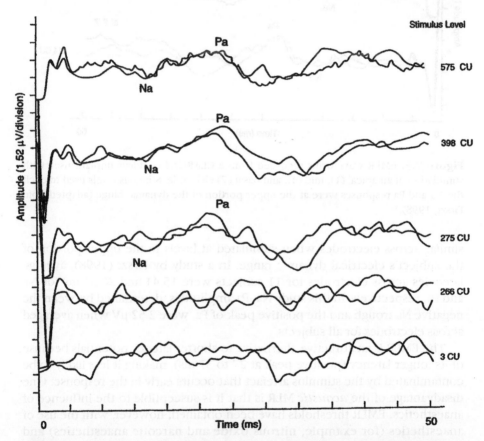

Figure 7.6. EMLR waveforms recorded from a CLARION cochlear implant user on electrode 4. Two recordings are shown for each stimulus current level between 575 clinical units (CU) and threshold. The Na–Pa complex is identifiable at higher stimulus levels, and threshold was 275 CU. No response is evident at 266 CU. A control run was recorded at the lowest amplitude input (3 CU) generated by the stimulus software (adapted from Firszt, 1998).

CLARION cochlear implant user as stimulus level is decreased from a level that represents the upper portion of the electrical dynamic range to the MLR threshold. These characteristics suggest that the EMLR can be elicited reliably with a range of stimulus parameters and will have some elements in common with the acoustic MLR (for example, decrease in Na–Pa amplitude with subsequent decrease in stimulus level).

Studies of the electrical and acoustic MLR within the same subject suggest that both responses are activated by the same neural generators of the central system (Kileny et al., 1989). Figure 7.7 illustrates an intrasubject comparison of an acoustic MLR and an EMLR obtained from a patient undergoing

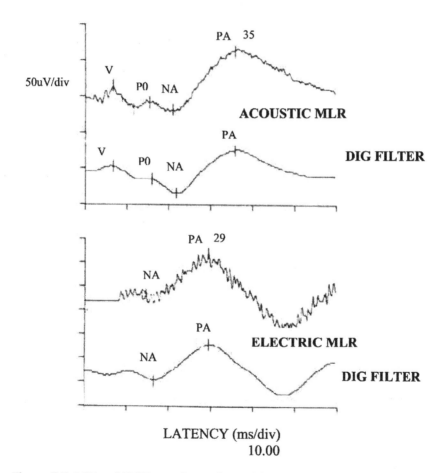

Figure 7.7. MLR and EMLR waveforms obtained from the normally hearing and deaf ear respectively of the same subject. The lower traces in each case have been digitally filtered (Figure 1 in Kileny et al., 1989).

labyrinthectomy to treat intractable Ménière's disease. The acoustic MLR was obtained by stimulating the normally hearing ear with an 85 dB click. The EMLR was obtained by stimulating the patient's contralateral deaf ear with biphasic electrical pulses prior to undertaking the operative procedure. Both responses were recorded after the establishment of general anaesthesia with fentanyl or sufentanil and nitrous oxide. The main difference between the acoustic MLR and its electrical counterpart is that, as expected, the latency of the Pa peak is reduced in the electrical mode relative to the acoustic mode (in this case, the difference was 6 ms).

Studies of the effects of temporal lobe lesions on the acoustic MLR suggest the Pa component is associated with the auditory temporal cortex (Kraus et al., 1982; Kileny et al., 1987), so the EMLR should also reflect cortical auditory centres important for speech understanding. It is plausible that variation in speech perception performance between subjects may be associated with higher cortical levels that involve the generators responsible for the MLR. In a study by Firszt et al. (2002a), variability in speech perception scores of cochlear implant recipients was related to neurophysiological responses at higher cortical levels. These findings were demonstrated with EMLR responses. Among 11 tested subjects, three subjects with no open set speech perception demonstrated an absence of the MLR response on all tested electrodes. Figure 7.8 shows EMLR responses for three subjects who had open set word understanding (S6, S7 and S11) and three subjects with no EMLR responses who scored 0% on all open set test measures (S4, S8 and S9) (Firszt, 1998).

In a study by Groenen et al. (2000) with 12 deaf adults using the Nucleus® device, EMLR amplitude variation (Na to Pa, Nb to Pb) across electrode sites (electrodes 20, 15, 10, 5, and 1) was reported to relate to suprasegmental speech understanding. In addition, EMLR interlatency variation was related to segmental speech processing. Poorer cochlear implant users had greater variation in amplitude and interlatency measures for the main components of the EMLR compared to better cochlear implant performers.

Animal studies suggest that EMLR measures correlate with neural survival (Jyung et al., 1989). It has also been proposed that the EMLR may be useful as both an indicator of eighth nerve survival in humans (Gardi, 1985) and to determine efficacy of electrical stimulation in an animal model (Burton et al., 1989). Figure 7.9 shows guinea pig EMLR amplitude/intensity functions obtained with different sites of electrical stimulation. The amplitude/intensity function obtained with modiolar stimulation (M) demonstrates the lowest threshold at 38 µA and a rapid saturation in growth function. For the scala tympani stimulation site, (ST) the threshold was 275 µA and the saturation was equally steep to modiolar stimulation but at a different current level.

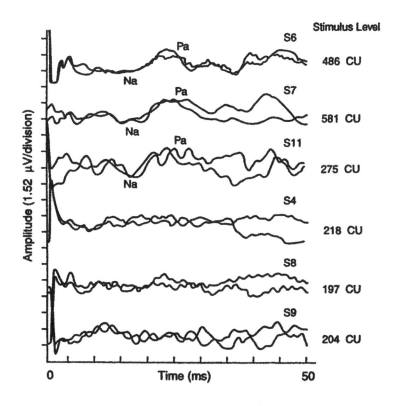

Figure 7.8. EMLR waveforms obtained from six subjects on an apical electrode of the CLARION cochlear implant. The stimulus level that represented the upper portion of the electrical dynamic range used to elicit responses is displayed for each subject. Note the lack of responses for subjects 4, 8, and 9 who scored 0% on open set speech perception measures (adapted from Figure 6 in Firszt et al., 2002a).

The highest threshold was appreciated with round window (RW) stimulation (500 µA) and the amplitude increase was much more gradual than at any of the other sites. As one of the main efforts in cochlear implant development is successful modiolar proximity of the electrode array, these studies suggest that the measurement of middle latency potentials in animal models is of particular importance.

Cortical auditory evoked potentials

Acoustic stimulation

The long latency or cortical auditory evoked potentials (AEPs) are believed to be most sensitive to disorders that may occur or originate in the central

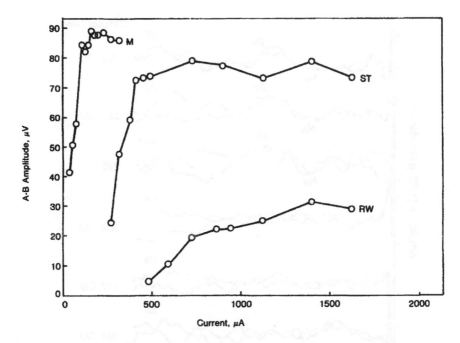

Figure 7.9. EMLR amplitude/intensity functions recorded from a guinea pig with electrical stimulation delivered at three sites: round window (RW); scala tympani (ST); and modiolus (M). (Figure 3 in Burton et al., 1989.)

auditory pathways. The most studied cortical AEPs include P1 (also referred to as Pb of the MLR), N1, P2, N2, MMN, P300 and N400. In general, these potentials are affected less by stimulus characteristics, such as frequency or duration, and more by elements of the task and subject factors, including attention. The late potentials reflect activity that is central to the brainstem and involve multiple structures that integrate sensory input types including auditory, visual and somatosensory stimuli (Davis, 1939; Näätänen and Picton, 1987).

The N1-P2 complex was first described by Davis (1939). The N1 wave is thought to consist of three distinct components, as reported by Näätänen and Picton (1987), and is affected by the temporal properties of the stimulus, subject state, and subject age. In the adult, N1 is a negative wave that occurs at approximately 100 ms after an auditory stimulus is initiated and is largest when recorded at the vertex. N1 is preceded by P1 with a latency of approximately 50 ms and smaller amplitude. P2 follows N1 as a positive peak with a latency of approximately 200 ms, and also is elicited with a repetitive identical stimulus. There are documented changes in P1-N1 responses in children. In studies of normally hearing children, P1 latency and amplitude decreases occur up to the age of 20 years (Ponton et al., 1996a; Sharma et al., 1997). Children may also demonstrate a negative wave that separates two positive peaks with significant decreases in latency with age. In summary, N1 components are thought to have both different source locations and times of development, although they stabilize by adolescence (Goodin et al., 1978; Martin et al., 1988; Courchesne, 1990).

Different components of the N1 depend on the stimulus features. For example, when a deviant stimulus is presented in a train of identical stimuli, N1 is still present but additionally a second negative wave occurs, the mismatch negativity or MMN (Näätänen et al., 1978). N1, P2 and N2 are elicited by stimulus onset and repetition, and are sensitive to stimulus parameters such as rate (Davis et al., 1966; Picton et al., 1981) and rise-fall time (Kodera et al., 1979). With decreased stimulus intensity, N1 amplitude decreases and latency increases (Picton et al., 1977). N1 amplitude has been found to decrease with a corresponding increase in frequency, especially those greater than 2,000 Hz. The N1-P2 complex has been shown to reflect changes in neural activity, such as increased N1-P2 symmetry in subjects with unilateral hearing loss (Ponton et al., 2001) and increased N1-P2 amplitude in normally hearing subjects after listening training (Tremblay et al., 2001).

In addition, N1 has good correspondence with behavioural thresholds and has been used as a tool to assist with assessment of hearing (Davis and Zerlin, 1966; Keidel, 1976). Studies have looked at the N1 response with both tones and speech stimuli. Lawson and Gaillard (1981) measured N1 elicited with tonal stimuli and consonant-vowel (CV) syllables that varied in duration. There was no difference reported when N1 was recorded with either tones or short durational consonant speech stimuli. In another study by Woods and Elmasian (1986), N1 was elicited with speech and tones, and the result was a similarity in the scalp distribution for either stimulus. Both studies suggest similar neural processes for tonal and phonetic stimuli when measured with the N1 evoked potential.

With acoustic stimulation and in the case of abnormal neural synchrony, the presence of late auditory potentials does not necessarily accompany normal earlier potentials (Starr et al., 1991; Berlin et al., 1993; Kraus et al., 1993a). Likewise, a normal early potential does not guarantee normal responses beyond the brainstem. Auditory evoked responses from more than one level of the pathway are important for complete understanding of auditory system function.

Cortical AEP neural generators

The generators of the cortical auditory responses are not as well understood as those of the earlier potentials. They appear to arise from wider ranging areas including the auditory cortex and the association areas. The temporal lobes and the limbic system are known to have great involvement with the late potentials (Kraus and McGee, 1992). According to Scherg et al. (1989), who used dipole source analysis, and other researchers studying intracerebral recordings, the N1 components may have three auditory cortex sources. N1 is believed to arise from a superior temporal cortex generator (Vaughan and Ritter, 1970; Näätänen, 1984). A second N1 subcomponent may be generated by the auditory cortex on the supratemporal plane (Celesia, 1976; McCallum and Curry, 1979; Perrault and Picton, 1984). A third N1 subcomponent probably originates from the association auditory cortex and the superior temporal gyrus (temporal and parietal cortex) (Hari et al., 1982; Velasco et al., 1985). It is also thought that activity from the motor and premotor cortices are involved with N1. P2 has generators in the auditory cortex (Vaughan and Ritter, 1970; Hari et al., 1980; Elberling et al., 1982), and N2 has involvement with the subcortical limbic generators (Näätänen et al., 1982).

Electrical stimulation

Cortical responses provide a mechanism for understanding how electrical stimuli are registered by the central auditory system of profoundly hearing-impaired individuals. There have been a limited number of studies during the past 10 years concerned with electrical late potentials and cochlear implant users. It is suggested that differences in subject performance may be due to differences in the central auditory system. Late potentials used for this purpose have included the N1, P2, P300 and MMN response elicited with tonal stimuli (Oviatt and Kileny, 1991), stimulated electrodes (Ponton and Don, 1995; Ponton et al., 1996a and 1996b; Firszt, 1998), and speech (Kaga et al., 1991; Kraus et al., 1993b; Micco et al., 1995). Several studies suggest that cortical responses can be reliably recorded with electrical stimulation.

Figure 7.10 illustrates N1–P2 responses elicited from an apical, medial and basal electrode of a CLARION cochlear implant user. These recordings and those from other subjects (Firszt, 1998) suggest that the N1–P2 waveforms are similar in morphology across electrodes within subjects. Mean latency across electrodes when stimulated at upper portions of the electrical dynamic range were 86 ms for N1 and 181 ms for P2 in a group of CLARION cochlear implant users (Firszt, 1998). These latencies may be slightly earlier than the acoustic counterpart for each component, depending on the comparison study's subject sample and stimulus characteristics. In a study by Ponton and Don (1995) with both normally hearing subjects and Nucleus CI22M cochlear implant users, the mismatch negativity (MMN) was elicited by either acoustic or electrical click stimuli that differed in duration or pitch. For both stimuli, the peak latencies (N1 and the MMN difference wave) for

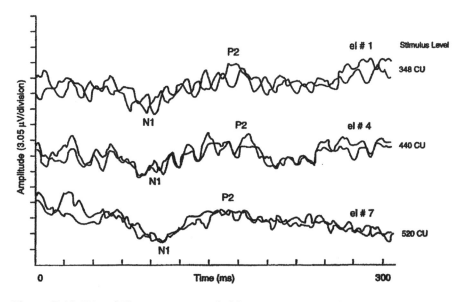

Figure 7.10. N1 and P2 responses recorded from a CLARION cochlear implant user with stimulation of an apical (1), mid (4) and basal (7) electrode. Stimulus levels used to elicit the N1 and P2 responses were at the upper portion of the dynamic range (adapted from Firszt, 1998).

the implant subjects were earlier (10 to 20 ms) than the responses for the normally hearing subjects.

N1-P2 amplitude measures have been reported for CLARION cochlear implant users as 5.65 µV, 4.78 µV, and 3.85 µV for electrodes 1 (apical), 4 (mid), and 7 (basal), respectively (Firszt, 1998). The effects of decreasing stimulus level on the N1-P2 response are shown in Figure 7.11. Five tracings from an individual subject recorded at decreasing stimulus levels show that amplitude measures decrease as electrical stimulus level (represented in clinical units, CU) decreases.

Oviatt and Kileny (1991) studied 10 Nucleus subjects and presented tone pairs in an oddball paradigm (500 Hz as the frequent stimulus, either 1,000, 2,000 or 3,000 Hz as the rare stimulus). For these subjects, N1 and P2 responses were identified with a 500 Hz stimulus, and P300 was present in at least nine of the 10 subjects for all three contrasts (500-1,000 Hz, 500-2,000 Hz, 500-3,000 Hz). In this study with tonal stimuli, P300 latencies were significantly longer in cochlear implant users than age-matched controls. It is well known in studies with acoustic stimulation that P300 latency increases as the task becomes more difficult (Duncan-Johnson and Donchin, 1982; Squires and Hecox, 1983). Discrimination of tones is a more difficult task for cochlear implant users compared to subjects with normal hearing.

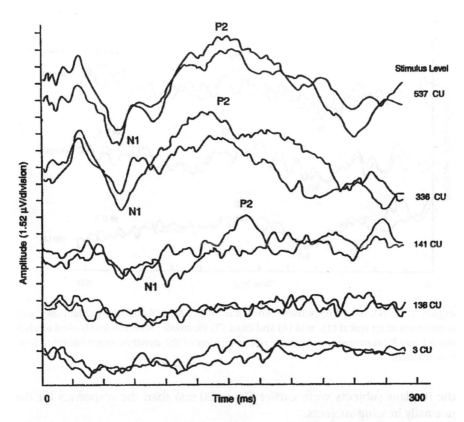

Figure 7.11. N1 and P2 responses recorded from a CLARION cochlear implant user at various stimulus levels. N1 and P2 are identifiable at stimulus levels that range from 537 CU to threshold, 141 CU. No response is obtained at 136 CU or during the control run of 3 CU (adapted from Firszt, 1998).

Micco et al. (1995) studied late potentials in Nucleus cochlear implant subjects who were instructed to listen for computer-generated speech stimuli. N1, P2 and P300 results were reported for 10 Nucleus implant users and age-matched hearing controls. There were no significant differences between the two groups with respect to latencies of N1, N2, or P300. N1 amplitude was reported to be smaller for subjects implanted with Nucleus devices. It may be that discrimination of speech is not as difficult as discrimination of tones for cochlear implant subjects, accounting for the longer P300 latencies noted by Oviatt and Kileny (1991).

Figure 7.12 displays electrical N1 and P2 responses for six subjects described in Firszt et al. (2002a). Subjects 4 and 9 had no N1–P2 responses when stimulated through their cochlear implant devices. These same two subjects did not demonstrate EMLRs, as noted earlier. Subject 8 had an N1–P2

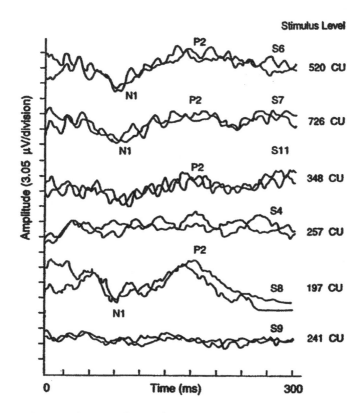

Figure 7.12. N1 and P2 waveforms obtained from six subjects with a CLARION cochlear implant. Four of the six subjects have identifiable responses at levels that were in the upper portion of the electrical dynamic range for the subject. Two subjects have no responses: S4 and S9 (adapted from Figure 7 in Firszt et al., 2001a).

response on selected electrodes tested, even though there were no EMLRs, as seen in Figure 7.8. According to Näätänen (1990), the presence of N1 indicates conscious detection of an auditory stimulus, rather than discrimination of stimuli. This is evident in studies, for example, of the MMN in which changes in the MMN latency occur with varying degrees of deviance in the stimuli but there is no difference in the N1 latency (Sams et al., 1985; Näätänen and Picton, 1987). With a repetitive stimulus, the presence of the N1 and P2 components may provide information about the integrity of the system to detect electrical stimuli, but may not be associated with word discrimination ability. A similar finding has been reported in a study with normally hearing subjects (Whiting et al., 1998) in which N1, N2, and P3 cortical evoked responses were investigated under varying conditions of decreased audibility using broadband noise masking. The N1 remained identifiable even when N2 and P3 were absent and when the subject could not discriminate the stimuli in the behavioural task. These results in normally hearing subjects are generally consistent with those studies reported by other researchers in which subjects are using cochlear implants.

The late evoked potential may serve as an indication that the subject has detected the signal (N1, P2) and the cognitive evoked potential (P3, MMN) may be used as an indicator of discrimination or contrast perception. Figure 7.13 illustrates N1–P2–P3 (P300, lower trace) and P3B (upper trace) components obtained from a nine-year-old patient with 'good' cochlear implant performance. Figure 7.14 illustrates N1–P2 components (both upper trace for the frequent stimuli and lower trace for the rare stimuli) for an individual subject. There is no well-defined P3 or P300 peak in this recording from a 12-year-old who was considered to be a 'poor' performer with a cochlear implant. Poor speech recognition performance (0% on open set speech tests) correlated with an absence of the cognitive component of the late auditory evoked potential.

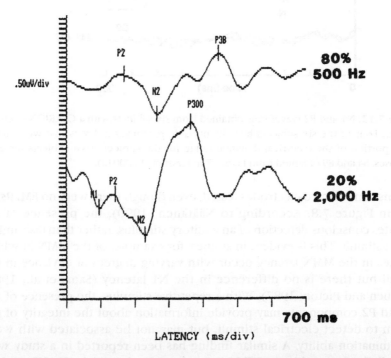

Figure 7.13. Late and cognitive auditory evoked potentials obtained from a nine-year-old subject with a cochlear implant. The stimuli consisted of 500 Hz (frequent) and 2,000 Hz (rare) tonebursts delivered in the soundfield at 70 dBSPL while the subject listened passively.

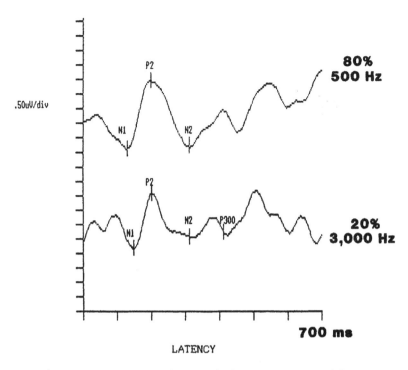

Figure 7.14. Late and cognitive auditory evoked potentials obtained from a 12-year-old subject with a cochlear implant. The stimuli consisted of 500 Hz (frequent) and 3,000 Hz (rare) tonebursts delivered in the soundfield at 70 dBSPL while the subject listened passively. The subject could detect both sets of stimuli well but could not distinguish between the frequent and the rare.

One advantage of the cortical auditory evoked potential is the ability to obtain these responses using speech stimuli. Figure 7.15 demonstrates N1–P2 components from a prelingually deaf adult patient with six years of cochlear implant experience in response to vowel–consonant–vowel stimuli (AMA upper trace and ASA lower trace). The presence of these responses to speech stimuli provides information regarding auditory and association cortex activation in this patient with long-term preimplant auditory deprivation. These responses (along with cognitive evoked responses) may be a suitable tool for longitudinal monitoring of neurophysiological progress in prelingually deaf, implanted patients.

Cortical potentials may reflect both degeneration and remaining plasticity of the auditory system of those with profound hearing loss receiving implant devices. Recent studies by Ponton and colleagues have incorporated electrically evoked potentials to study maturation of cortical auditory function in children. Studies indicate that latency changes for P1 occur at the same rate

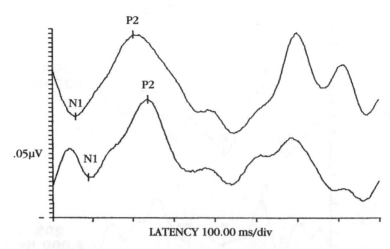

Figure 7.15. N1 and P2 responses recorded from an adult with six years' cochlear implant experience. The stimulus was a VCV nonsense syllable delivered in the soundfield at 70 dBSPL.

for normally hearing children as for children with cochlear implants, but the overall maturation sequence is delayed. Additionally, the delay period for the electrophysiologic response corresponds with the length of auditory deprivation (Ponton et al., 1996a and 1996b). Findings from Ponton and colleagues suggest that the auditory system needs stimulation to mature, and that when electrical stimulation is introduced via cochlear implantation, the system resumes maturation. The mismatch negativity, or MMN, has been shown to be present in good cochlear implant users and may be a better measure of auditory system development needed to acquire high levels of speech perception (Ponton et al., 2000).

In summary, N1 may not relate to discrimination of speech stimuli, but instead represents an obligatory response reflecting the presence of the stimuli. It appears that cortical responses could provide insight into how the central system detects and discriminates signals from the implant. While a number of recent studies cite the central auditory pathway as a potential source that may influence subject outcomes (Ponton et al., 1996a and 1996b; Cunningham et al., 2000; Ponton et al., 2000; Firszt et al., 2002a; Tremblay et al., 2001) it has been predominantly overlooked in studies of cochlear implant recipients.

Conclusion

This chapter provided an overview of clinical and experimental applications of middle and late auditory potentials obtained with extracochlear or intracochlear electrical stimulation. There are several advantages associated with these electrophysiological responses to electrically mediated auditory stimulation. First, both late and middle latency responses have a relatively long latency and therefore are not prone to distortion or even obliteration by the electrical stimulus artefact. Second, the presence of a middle latency or late electrically evoked response indicates that the auditory pathway is activated by electrical stimulation to the level of the auditory cortex. Thus when obtaining one of these responses from an implanted patient, especially from one with relatively poor performance, the assumption can be made that the patient has at least detected the stimulus. Furthermore, as shown by recent work of one of the authors (JBF), middle latency responses may also be associated with some perceptual correlates, not just detection. Thus, in order to confirm electrical excitability and at least detection of electrical-auditory stimulation by an implant user (or preimplant, with transtympanic promontory stimulation) clinicians should consider the electrically evoked MLR or cortical AEP, unless it is not feasible due to the age of the patient or anaesthetic considerations. The late response is not suitable under anaesthesia, but as shown in this chapter, with special techniques, the MLR can be obtained under anaesthesia. These considerations also belong to the list of disadvantages of late and middle latency potentials. If anaesthesia or sedation are necessary, the electrically evoked compound action potential (ECAP) or the EABR would be the responses of choice. Another disadvantage particular to the MLR is that it is unpredictable in young children, unless sleep stage is carefully monitored. In most clinical settings, that is not always feasible. The late evoked response is present at a very young age, but it is important to be familiar with the effects of maturational changes on the response. Both the MLR and the cortical AEP are affected by state, in particular during Stage 4 sleep.

Overall, both the electrically evoked MLR and cortical AEP can be useful components in the clinical management of the implanted patient or the cochlear implant candidate. It is expected that clinicians and researchers will continue to study the middle and late latency responses to further our understanding of auditory function with electrical stimulation.

Acknowledgements

We wish to thank Dr Ron Chambers for editorial comments on portions of this manuscript and Wolfgang Gaggl for technical assistance.

References

Abbas PJ (1993) Electrophysiology. In Tyler RS (ed.) Cochlear Implants: Audiological Foundations. San Diego: Singular Publishing Group.

Berlin C, Hood L, Cecola RP, Jackson D, Szabo P (1993) Afferent–efferent disconnection in humans. Hear Res 65: 40–50.

Brown CJ (1996) Using electrically evoked auditory potentials in the clinical management of cochlear implant candidates and recipients. Semin Hear 17 (4): 389–402.

Buchwald JS, Hinman C, Norman RS, Huang CM, Brown KA (1981) Middle and long latency auditory evoked potentials recorded from the vertex of normal and chronically lesioned cats. Brain Res 205: 91–109.

Burton NJ, Miller JM, Kileny PR (1989) Middle latency responses: I. Electrical and acoustic stimulation. Arch Otolaryngol 115: 59–62.

Cacace AT, Satya-Murti S, Wolpaw JR (1990) Human middle-latency auditory evoked potentials: vertex and temporal components. Electroencephalogr Clin Neurophysiol 77: 6–18.

Celesia GG (1976) Organization of auditory cortical areas in man. Brain 99: 403–14.

Chambers RD (1992) Differential age effects for components of the adult auditory middle latency response. Hear Res 58: 123–31.

Chambers RD, Griffiths SK (1991) Effects of age on the adult auditory middle latency response. Hear Res 51: 1–10.

Courchesne E (1990) Chronology of postnatal brain development: event-related potential, positron emission tomography, myelinogenesis and synaptogenesis studies. In Rohrbaugh J, Parasuraman R, Johnson R (eds.) Event-related Brain Potentials. New York: Oxford University Press.

Cunningham J, Nicol T, Zecker S, Kraus N (2000) Speech evoked neurophysiologic responses in children with learning problems: development and behavioral correlates of perception. Ear Hear 21: 554–68.

Davis H, Mast T, Yoshie N, Zerlin S (1966) The slow response of the human cortex to auditory stimuli: recovery process. Electroencephalogr Clin Neurophysiol 21: 105–13.

Davis H, Zerlin S (1966) Acoustic relations of the human vertex potential. J Ac Soc Am 39: 109–16.

Davis PA (1939) Effects of acoustic stimuli on the waking human brain. J Neurophysiol 2: 494–9.

Duncan-Johnson C, Donchin E (1982) The P300 component of the event-related brain potential as an index of information processing. Biol Psychol 14: 1–52.

Elberling C, Bak C, Kofoed B, Lebech J, Saermark K (1982) Auditory magnetic fields from the human cerebral cortex: location and strength of an equivalent current dipole. Acta Neurol Scand 65: 553–69.

Firszt JB (1998) Electrically evoked auditory potentials recorded at three levels of the auditory pathway from multichannel cochlear implant subjects: characterization and comparison to behavioral levels. Doctoral dissertation, University of Illinois, Champaign-Urbana.

Firszt JB, Chambers RD, Kraus N (2002a) Neurophysiology of cochlear implant users II: comparison among speech perception, dynamic range and physiological measures. Ear Hear (submitted).

Firszt JB, Chambers RD, Kraus N, Reeder RM (2002b) Neurophysiology of cochlear implant users I: effects of stimulus current level and electrode site on the ABR, MLR, and N1-P2 response. Ear Hear (submitted).

Firszt JB, Rotz LA, Chambers RD, Novak MA (1999) Electrically evoked potentials recorded in adult and pediatric Clarion implant users. Ann Otol Rhinol Laryngol Suppl 177: 58–63.

Gardi JN (1985) Human brainstem and middle latency responses to electrical stimulation: preliminary observations. In Schindler RA, Merzenich MM (eds) Cochlear Implants. New York: Raven Press, pp. 351–63.

Goldstein R, Rodman LB (1967) Early components of averaged evoked responses to rapidly repeated auditory stimuli. J Speech Hear Res 10: 697-705.

Goodin DS, Squires KC, Henderson BH, Starr A (1978) Age-related variations in evoked potentials to auditory stimuli in normal human subjects. Electroencephalogr Clin Neurophysiol 44: 447-58.

Groenen P, Makhdoum M, Snik A, Van den Broek P (2000) Auditory middle latency responses and speech perception in cochlear implant users. In Waltzman S, Cohen N (eds) Cochlear Implants. New York: Thieme Medical Publishers, pp. 134-5.

Hari R, Aittoniemi K, Jarvinen ML, Katila T, Varpula T (1980) Auditory evoked transient and sustained magnetic fields of the human brain. Exp Brain Res 40: 237-40.

Hari R, Kaila K, Katila T, Tuomisto T, Varpula T (1982) Interstimulus interval dependence of the auditory vertex response and its magnetic counterpart: implications for their neural generation. Electroencephalogr Clin Neurophysiol 54: 561-9.

Ho KJ, Kileny PR, Paccioretti D, McLean, DR (1987) Neurologic, audiologic and electrophysiologic sequelae of bilateral temporal lobe lesions. Arch Neurol 44: 982-7.

Jacobson JT (1985) Normative aspects of the pediatric auditory brainstem response. J Otolaryngol 14: 5-6.

Jyung RW, Miller JM, Cannon SC (1989) Evaluation of eighth nerve integrity by the electrically evoked middle latency response. Otolaryngol Head Neck Surg101: 670-82.

Kaga K, Kodera K, Hirota E, Tsuzuka T (1991) P300 response to tones and speech sounds after cochlear implant: a case report. Laryngoscope 101: 905-7.

Keidel WD (1976) The physiological background of the electric response audiometry. In Neff WD, Keidel WD (eds) Handbook of Sensory Physiology. Berlin, Heidelberg, New York: Springer-Verlag, pp. 105-231.

Kileny PR (1983) Auditory middle latency responses: current issues. Semin Hear 4: 403-13.

Kileny PR, Kemink JL (1987) Electrically evoked middle latency potentials in cochlear implant candidates. Arch Otolaryngol Head Neck Surg 113: 1072-7.

Kileny PR, Kemink JL, Miller JM (1989) An intrasubject comparison of electric and acoustic middle latency responses. Am J Otol 10(1): 23-7.

Kileny PR, Paccioretti D, Wilson AF (1987) Effects of cortical lesions on middle-latency auditory evoked responses (MLR). Electroencephalogr Clin Neurophysiol 66: 108-20.

Kileny PR, Shea S (1986) Middle-latency and 40 Hz auditory evoked responses in normal-hearing subjects: click and 500-Hz thresholds. J Speech Hear Res 29: 20-8.

Kodera, K, Hink RF, Yamada O, Suzuki J (1979) Effects of rise time on simultaneously recorded auditory-evoked potentials from the early, middle, and late ranges. Audiology 18: 395-402.

Kraus N, McGee T (1992) Electrophysiology of the human auditory system. In Popper AN, Fay RR (eds) The Mammalian Auditory Pathway: Neurophysiology. New York: Springer-Verlag.

Kraus N, McGee T, Comperatore C (1989) MLRs in children are consistently present during wakefulness, stage I and REM sleep. Ear Hear 10: 339-45.

Kraus N, McGee T, Ferre J, Hoeppner J, Carrell T, Sharma A, Nicol T (1993a) Mismatch negativity in the neurophysiologic/behavioral evaluation of auditory processing deficits: a case study. Ear Hear 14(4): 223-34.

Kraus N, Micco AG, Koch DB, McGee T, Carrell T, Sharma A, Wiet RJ, Weingarten CZ (1993b) The mismatch negativity cortical evoked potential elicited by speech in cochlear-implant users. Hear Res 65: 118-24.

Kraus N, Özdamar O, Hier D, Stein L (1982) Auditory middle latency responses (MLRs) in patients with cortical lesions. Electroencephalogr Clin Neurophysiol 54: 274–87.

Kraus N, Smith D, McGee T (1987) Rate and filter effects on the developing middle latency response. Audiology 26: 257–68.

Kraus N, Smith D, McGee T (1988) Midline and temporal lobe MLRs in guinea pig originate from different generators: a conceptual framework for new and existing data. Electroencephalogr Clin Neurophysiol 00: 1–18.

Kraus N, Smith D, Reed N, Stein L, Cartree C (1985) Auditory middle latency responses in children: effects of age and diagnostic category. Electroencephalogr Clin Neurophysiol 62: 343–51.

Lawson E, Gaillard A (1981) Evoked potentials to consonant-vowel syllables. Acta Psychol 49: 17–25.

Littman T, Kraus N, McGee T, Nicol T (1992) Binaural stimulation reveals functional differences between midline and temporal components of the MLR in the guinea pig. Electroencephalogr Clin Neurophysiol 84: 362–72.

Martin L, Barajas J, Fernandez R, Torres E (1988) Auditory event-related potentials in well characterized groups of children. Electroencephalogr Clin Neurophysiol 71: 375–81.

McCallum WC, Curry SH (1979) Hemisphere differences in event related potentials and CNVs associated with monaural stimuli and lateralized motor responses. In Lehmann D, Callaway E (eds) Human Evoked Potentials: Applications and Problems. New York: Plenum, pp. 235–50.

McGee TJ, Kraus N, Comperatore C, Nicol T (1991) Subcortical and cortical components of the MLR generating system. Brain Res 544: 211–20.

McGee T, Kraus N, Killion M, Rosenberg R, King C (1993) Improving the reliability of the auditory middle latency response by monitoring EEG delta activity. Ear Hear 14: 76–84.

McGee T, Kraus N, Littman T, Nicol T (1992) Contributions of medial geniculate body subdivisions to the middle latency response. Hear Res 61: 147–54.

Mendel MI, Kupperman GL (1974) Early components of the averaged electroencephalic response to constant level clicks during rapid eye movement sleep. Audiology 13: 23–32.

Micco AG, Kraus N, Koch DB, McGee TJ, Carrell TD, Sharma A, Nicol T, Wiet RJ (1995) Speech-evoked cognitive P300 potentials in cochlear implant recipients. Am J Otol 16(4): 514–20.

Miyamoto RT (1986) Electrically evoked potentials in cochlear implant subjects. Laryngoscope 96: 178–85.

Musiek FE, Geurkink NA (1981) Auditory brainstem and middle latency evoked response sensitivity near threshold. Ann Otol 90: 236–40.

Näätänen R (1984) In search of a short-duration memory trace of a stimulus in human brain. In Pulkkinen L, Lyytinen L (eds) Essays in Honour of Martti Takala, Jyvaskyla Studies in Education, Psychology, and Social Science. Jyvaskyla: University of Jyvaskyla.

Näätänen R (1990) The role of attention in auditory information processing as revealed by event-related brain potentials and other brain measures of cognitive function. Behav Brain Res 13: 201–33.

Näätänen R, Gaillard AWK, Mantysalo S (1978) Early selective attention effect on evoked potential reinterpreted. Acta Psychol 42: 313–29.

Näätänen R, Picton T (1987) The N1 wave of the human electric and magnetic response to sound: a review and an analysis of the component structure. Psychophysiol 24: 375-425.

Näätänen R, Simpson M, Loveless NE (1982) Stimulus deviance and evoked potentials. Biol Psychol 14: 53-98.

National Institutes of Health (NIH) (1995) Cochlear implants in adults and children. Consensus Development Conference Statement 13 (2).

Osterhammel PA, Shallop JK, Terkildsen K (1985) The effect of sleep on the auditory brainstem response (ABR) and the middle latency response (MLR). Scand Audiol 14: 47-50.

Oviatt DL, Kileny PR (1991) Auditory event-related potentials elicited from cochlear implant recipients and hearing subjects. Am J Audiol 1: 48-55.

Özdamar O, Kraus N (1983) Auditory middle latency responses in humans. Audiology 22: 34-49.

Perrault N, Picton TW (1984) Event-related potentials recorded from the scalp and nasopharynx. I. N1 and P2. Electroencephalogr Clin Neurophysiol 59: 177-94.

Picton TW, Hillyard SA, Krausz HI, Galambos R (1974) Human auditory evoked potentials. I. Evaluation of components. Electroencephalogr Clin Neurophysiol 36: 179-90.

Picton TW, Stapells DR, Campbell KB (1981) Auditory evoked potentials from the human cochlea and brainstem. J Otolaryngol 10: 1-14.

Picton TW, Woods DL, Baribeau-Braun J, Healey TM (1977) Evoked potential audiometry. J Otolaryngol 6: 90-119.

Ponton CW, Don M (1995) The mismatch negativity in cochlear implant users. Ear Hear 16(1): 130-46.

Ponton CW, Don M, Eggermont JJ, Waring MD, Masuda A (1996a) Maturation of human cortical auditory function: differences between normal hearing and cochlear implant children. Ear Hear 17: 430-7.

Ponton CW, Don M, Eggermont JJ, Waring MD, Kwong B, Masuda A (1996b) Auditory system plasticity in children after long periods of complete deafness. Neuroreport 8: 61-5.

Ponton CW, Don M, Eggermont JJ, Waring MD, Kwong B, Cunningham J, Trautwein P (2000) Maturation of the mismatch negativity: effects of profound deafness and cochlear implant use. Aud Neuro-Otol 5: 167-85.

Ponton CW, Vasama JP, Tremblay K, Khosla D, Kwong B, Don M (2001) Plasticity in the adult human central auditory system: evidence from late-onset profound unilateral deafness. Hear Res 154 (1-2): 32-44.

Sams M, Paavilainen P, Alho K, Näätänen R (1985) Auditory frequency discrimination and event-related potentials. Electroencephalogr Clin Neurophysiol 62: 437-48.

Scherg M (1982) Distortion of the middle latency auditory response produced by analog filtering. Scand Audiol 11: 57-60.

Scherg M, Hari R, Hanalainen M (1990) Frequency specific sources of the auditory N19-P30-P50 responses detected by a multiple source analysis of evoked magnetic fields and potentials. In Williamson S (ed.) Advances in Biomagnetism. New York: Plenum Press.

Scherg M, Vajsar J, Picton T (1989) A source analysis of the late human auditory evoked potentials. J Cogn Neurosci 1: 336-55.

Scherg M, Volk SA (1983) Frequency specificity of simultaneously recorded early and middle latency auditory evoked potentials. Electroencephalogr Clin Neurophysiol 56: 443-52.

Scherg M, Von Cramon D (1986) Evoked dipole source potentials of the human auditory cortex. Electroencephalogr Clin Neurophysiol 65: 344-60.

Shallop JK, Beiter AL, Goin DW, Mischke RE (1990) Electrically evoked auditory brainstem responses (EABR) and middle latency responses (EMLR) obtained from patients with the Nucleus multichannel cochlear implant. Ear Hear 11(1): 5-15.

Sharma A, Kraus N, McGee TJ, Nicol TG (1997) Developmental changes in P1 and N1 central auditory responses elicited by consonant-vowel syllables. Electroencephalogr Clin Neurophysiol 104(6): 540-5.

Simmons FB, Smith L (1983) Estimating nerve survival by electrical ABR. Ann N Y Acad Sci 405: 422-3.

Squires KC, Hecox KE (1983) Electrophysiological evaluation of higher level auditory processing. Semin Hear 4(4): 415-33.

Starr A, McPherson D, Patterson J, Luxford W, Shannon R, Sininger Y, Tonokawa L, Waring M (1991) Absence of both auditory evoked potentials and auditory percepts dependent on time cues. Brain 114: 1157-80.

Stein LK, Kraus N (1988) Auditory evoked potentials with special populations. Semin Hear 9: 35-45.

Suzuki T, Hirabayashi M, Kobayashi K (1984) Effects of analog and digital filtering on auditory middle latency responses in adults and young children. Ann Otol 93: 267-70.

Tremblay K, Kraus N, McGee T, Ponton C, Otis B (2001) Central auditory plasticity: changes in the N1-P2 complex after speech-sound training. Ear Hear 22: 79-90.

Van den Honert C, Stypulkowski PH (1986) Characterization of the electrically evoked auditory brainstem response (ABR) in cats and humans. Hear Res 21: 109-26.

Vaughan Jr HG, Ritter W (1970) The sources of auditory evoked responses recorded from the human scalp. Electroencephalogr Clin Neurophysiol 28: 360-7.

Velasco M, Velasco F, Olvera A (1985) Subcortical correlates of the somatic, auditory, and visual vertex activities in man. I. Bipolar EEG responses and electrical stimulation. Electroencephalogr Clin Neurophysiol 61: 519-29.

Walsh SN, Leake-Jones P (1982) Chronic electrical stimulation of auditory nerve in cat: physiological and histological results. Hear Res 7: 281-304.

Whiting KA, Martin BA, Stapells DR (1998) The effects of broadband noise masking on cortical event-related potentials to speech sounds /ba/ and /da/. Ear Hear 19: 218-31.

Woods DL, Clayworth CC (1986) Age-related changes in human middle latency auditory evoked potentials. Electroencephalogr Clin Neurophysiol 65: 297-303.

Woods D, Elmasian R (1986) The habituation of event-related potentials to speech sounds and tones. Electroencephalogr Clin Neurophysiol 65: 447-59.

CHAPTER 8

Cortical auditory evoked potentials recorded from cochlear implant users: methods and applications

CURTIS W PONTON, MANUEL DON

Contents

- Overview.
- Evoked potential generation from the brainstem to the cortex.
- Recording cortical AEPs from CI users: methodology.
- Recording the mismatch negativity.
- Review of cortical AEP studies with CI users.
- Conclusions.

Overview

For cochlear implant (CI) populations, auditory evoked potentials have primarily been used as measures of implant functionality by showing evidence of CI-driven auditory nerve and brainstem activity. However, the neurophysiological activity that follows auditory nerve and brainstem activity may also have an important role in clinical evaluation. These later auditory evoked potentials (cortical AEPs) reflect activation of the central nervous system pathways at the level of the thalamus and cortex. Cortical processes are essential for spoken language processing. As pointed out in Chapter 7, the AEPs that measure higher brain functions may have considerable value in understanding how deafness and CI use affect cortical processes that may be important for spoken language.

This chapter has three primary goals. The first is to review what is currently known about the generators underlying the cortical AEPs, as well as the relationship between certain AEPs and behavioural function. The second is to outline cortical AEP recording methodology. This will focus on general issues of data collection, as well as issues specific to acquiring cortical AEPs from CI users, namely dealing with the often-present stimulus artefact. This section will also review methods for recording and objectively detecting the mismatch negativity (MMN). These sections expand on topics described in Chapter 7, focusing more on the technical aspects of data acquisition and analysis of cortical AEPs. The third goal of this chapter is to review the results of cortical AEP studies of cochlear implant populations, with particular emphasis on data collected in the Electrophysiology Laboratory at the House Ear Institute.

Evoked potential generation from the brainstem to the cortex

For CI studies, the auditory nerve action potential and auditory brainstem response (ABR) have been the neurophysiological responses most used. The neural activity in these responses is contained in the time epoch covering the first 10 to 15 ms after stimulus onset. The ABR is considered to reflect synchronized action potentials generated along the ascending central auditory pathway from the level of the auditory nerve up to the level of the lateral lemniscus or perhaps the inferior colliculus (Møller and Jannetta, 1982). The amplitude of the ABR may be as large as 0.5 to 0.75 μV in normally hearing populations, and even larger in CI populations (up to 1 μV) due to more synchronous driving of the auditory nerve. In CI populations, the ABR has been used primarily as a measure of implant functionality (generating sufficient stimulation of the central auditory system to produce a synchronous neural response at the level of the brainstem). However, as noted by Abbas et al. (1999), the ABR may also be useful for determining whether the electrodes in a multichannel implant array activate distinct populations of auditory nerve fibres.

The cortical AEPs (also called event-related potentials) are distinguished from the ABR by longer latencies and larger amplitudes. Unlike the ABR, the amplitudes and latencies of the cortical AEPs are affected by a number of subject factors (for example state of arousal) or task demands. While the ABR primarily reflects synchronized action potentials, later AEPs mostly reflect postsynaptic potentials (PSPs) generated by commonly aligned (perpendicular to the cortical surface) cortical pyramidal cells (Creutzfeldt et al., 1966; Mitzdorf, 1986; Vaughan and Arezzo, 1988). Since approximately 85% of the connections in the cortex are excitatory, the AEPs predominantly reflect the activity of excitatory (EPSPs) rather than inhibitory (IPSPs) postsynaptic potentials (Steinschneider et al., 1994). Compared to the ABR, amplitudes of the later AEPs are much larger (ranging from 1 to 10.0 μV). As shown in Figure 8.1, these later AEPs, although much larger in amplitude than the ABR, are still much smaller than the background EEG (ranging from 10 μV up to

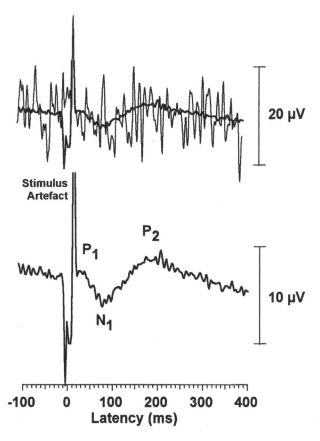

Figure 8.1. Cortical AEPs recorded from an adult CI user superimposed on a single sweep of EEG data. The stimulus artefact from the cochlear implant is clearly apparent. The amplitude of the background EEG (< 20 µV) for this subject is lower than that typically obtained from most subjects.

and exceeding 100 µV). Therefore, the cortical AEPs require the same signal averaging process as the ABR to be extracted from the background EEG.

The generator configuration underlying each peak of the cortical AEPs is more complex than that of the ABR. Each of the cortical AEP peaks typically represents activation of more than one neural generator (Vaughan and Arezzo, 1988). Moreover, auditory stimulation generates activity in at least three central nervous system pathways. These include two auditory system pathways (the lemniscal and lemniscal-adjunct pathways), as well as a non-specific multisensory pathway originating in the reticular activating system (RAS) (Graybiel, 1973; Weinberger, 1993). Thus, the cortical AEPs represent the sum of activity from these pathways that is of sufficient synchrony, magnitude and appropriate orientation to be recorded in the electrical far field by electrodes located on the scalp. Our understanding of the cortical AEP generators remains incomplete. However, a pathway-based model of cortical AEP generation will be outlined as a framework for understanding the origins of activity. This is summarized in Table 8.1 for the cortical AEPs shown in Figure 8.2.

Lemniscal pathway

The lemniscal pathway, which only responds to acoustic stimulation and is tonotopically organized, appears to code and register stimulus features. This pathway projects from the central nucleus of the inferior colliculus (ICc) to the ventral division of the medial geniculate nucleus (MGv), and terminates in layer IV of the primary auditory cortex (Weinberger and Diamond, 1987; Lennartz and Weinberger, 1992; Weinberger, 1993).

Auditory evoked potential peaks that contain components attributed to the lemniscal pathway include a late-maturing component of the middle latency response (MLR) peak Pa (Erwin and Buchwald, 1986a and 1986b;

Table 8.1. Pathway-based model of cortical AEP generation

	Lemniscal	Lemniscal-adjunct	RAS
Physiological features	Auditory-specific Tonotopically organized Early latency responses Time-locked	Not auditory specific Not tonotopically organized Broadly tuned	Multisensory
Anatomical pathway	ICc to MGv MGv to auditory primary	ICx to MGd and MGm MGd to auditory secondary MGm to all auditory areas	Mesencephalic reticular formation to reticular nucleus of the thalamus to the cortex
Initial cortical layer termination	Layer IV	MGd to layer IV (secondary cortex) MGm to layer I (all auditory)	All cortical layers
AEP peaks	Pa TP41, N1b	T-complex (Ta and Tb) MMN	Pa, Pb N1*, P2
Function	Registration of stimulus features	(Preattentive) discrimination	Modulatory Alerting

* Only for interstimulus intervals > 1–2 s

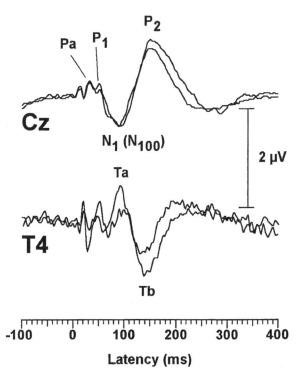

Figure 8.2. Cortical AEPs recorded from a normally hearing subject. The obligatory cortical AEPs (P1–N1–P2) are clearly represented at electrode Cz. The T-complex components Ta and Tb are the dominant AEPs present at electrode T4.

Kraus and McGee, 1993), as well as an N1 component labelled N1b (Näätänen and Picton, 1987). The Pa peak may represent the activity of two sources; one in the thalamus (MGv) and another in the primary auditory cortex (Scherg and von Cramon, 1986; Scherg et al., 1989; Cacace et al., 1990; Jacobson, 1994). The N1b is recorded maximally at fronto-central electrode locations. Lesion studies and source localization models suggest a bilateral superior temporal gyrus origin for N1b. The N1b is presumed to represent recurrent or re-entrant activation of the auditory cortex (Mäkelä and Hari, 1992; Mäkelä and McEvoy, 1996). Based on the work of individuals such as Kandel et al. (1991) and Steinschneider et al. (1994), it appears that N1b activity may originate from cortical layers II and upper III of the cortex.

Lemniscal-adjunct pathway

The lemniscal-adjunct pathway lacks a strong tonotopic organization and is not exclusively responsive to auditory stimulation. In behavioural conditioning studies using non-human mammals, it has been shown that this pathway may code the behavioural or psychological significance of a stimulus (Weinberger and Diamond, 1987; Weinberger, 1993). The lemniscal-adjunct pathway includes the external nucleus of the inferior colliculus (ICx), which projects to the dorsal (MGd) and medial (MGm) nuclei of the medial geniculate (Weinberger and Diamond, 1987; Weinberger, 1993). Afferents from the MGm terminate diffusely in layer I of all areas of the auditory cortex (including the secondary cortex), and then project to layers II and III (Winer, 1992). Afferents from the MGd terminate in layer IV of the secondary cortex (Lennartz and Weinberger, 1992) located on the lateral surface of the human temporal lobe.

Two AEP components that appear to reflect lemniscal-adjunct pathway activation are the T-complex and the MMN. The T-complex, so named because it is largest at scalp electrodes located over the temporal cortex, consists of two peaks: Ta, a positive peak that occurs at about 95 ms, and Tb (N1c), a negative peak that occurs at about 130 ms (Wolpaw and Penry, 1975; Giard et al., 1994). Dipole source models indicate that the T-complex origi-nates from the posterior lateral surface of the temporal lobe, which corre-sponds to the secondary auditory cortex (Scherg and von Cramon, 1986). Based on scalp electrode recordings, the T-complex is optimally recorded from more anterior temporal scalp locations, using electrodes in the vicinity of T3 and T4 (based on the International 10/20 system of electrode place-ment – Jasper, 1958). Activity recorded at more posterior temporal electrodes, for example, electrodes T5 and T6, is highly negatively correlated with activity recorded at electrodes C3 and C4. It is therefore likely that this activity represents activity of the opposite end of the current dipoles gener-ating the obligatory cortical AEPs (P1, N1, and P2) that are so robustly present at central and frontal electrodes approaching the midline of the head (Tonnquist-Uhlén et al., in press).

The MMN (which will be described in greater detail later in this chapter) is evoked using an oddball presentation sequence. In this sequence, a series of identical (standard) auditory stimuli is interspersed with a randomly placed, low probability, acoustically different (deviant) stimulus (Näätänen, 1990). A correlation has been demonstrated between the magnitude of the MMN and psychophysical discrimination thresholds in normally hearing populations. Thus, this response provides a neurophysiological estimate of perceived acoustic change (Kraus et al., 1996). In an animal model, Kraus et al. (1994) showed that a tone-evoked MMN-like response originates subcorti-cally in the lemniscal-adjunct caudomedial nucleus of the medial geniculate in the guinea pig. In humans, dipole source analysis studies suggest bilateral temporal generators in the auditory cortex anterior to the site of N1b generation (Näätänen and Michie, 1979; Scherg et al., 1989). A possible frontal source may contribute a late negativity to the MMN (Giard et al., 1990; Alho, 1995).

Reticular activating system (RAS) pathway

This pathway, which consists of the ascending reticular activating system and its thalamic projections, may serve as a modulatory or alerting mechanism (Graybiel, 1973; Weinberger, 1993). Buchwald et al. (1991) have strongly argued that activity along this pathway is a major source for the Pb of the MLR (often labelled P1 but likely a different component). Other AEP peaks that may originate from or be modulated by activity in this pathway are a fast maturing component of Pa (Kraus et al., 1994) and P2 (Rif et al., 1991). Several studies indicate that the RAS components contributing to the cortical AEP originate in the thalamus (Buchwald et al., 1991; Erwin et al., 1986b for Pb; Knight et al., 1980; Woods et al., 1993; Fischer et al., 1995 for P2), although the findings are not all in accord (Reite et al., 1988; Liégeois-Chauvel et al., 1994; Mäkelä et al., 1994). For P2, a thalamic source would be consistent with the suggestion of Rif et al. (1991) that this peak reflects the activity of a sensory gating process on the way to the auditory cortex at the level of the reticular nucleus of the thalamus (Skinner and Yingling, 1977; Yingling and Skinner, 1977).

In summary the cortical AEPs recorded from the scalp represent the activity of a complex generator system. This complexity makes interpretation of the cortical AEPs difficult, but not impossible. For the purposes of assessing spoken language processes in cochlear implant users, at least three AEPs are of particular interest:

- Presence of the N1 potential (specifically N1b), which dominates the obligatory cortical AEPs of normally hearing subjects, is considered to reflect the conscious detection of an auditory event (Hyde, 1997). ('Obligatory cortical AEPs' is a phrase commonly used to describe the P1–N1–P2 potentials, as the presentation of virtually any stimulus evokes these peaks.)
- The T-complex activity, recorded from electrodes located at anterior temporal scalp locations, has been associated with developmental language delays in normally hearing children (Tonnquist-Uhlén, 1996).
- For research purposes, the MMN (see later sections for figures) has become a commonly used measure of auditory short-term memory and discrimination processes, both of which are likely important prerequisites for spoken language processes. Moreover, the MMN may also have value as a measure of cortical plasticity (Tremblay et al., 1997; 1998).

Recording cortical AEPs from CI users: methodology

Under normal laboratory recording conditions (testing normally hearing young adults), obtaining good quality cortical AEPs can be challenging. Obtaining these from CI users not only presents the challenges of working with a clinical population, but also technical challenges due to the large electrical artefact produced by the implant hardware. This artefact persists at least as long as the implant is activated by stimulus input. Therefore, acquiring high quality cortical AEPs from individuals who use a cochlear implant can be more difficult than from non-CI clinical populations. Consequently, a number of methodological issues must be considered. Many of the issues described below apply to other electrically evoked potentials as well as the cortical AEPs.

Recording environment

A critical aspect in obtaining good quality cortical AEPs from any subject population is the quality of the recording environment. This is determined by several factors such as scalp electrode contact, stimulus artefact generated by the implant, and extraneous noise generated by the subject. Some of these factors are easily controlled, others may require considerable ingenuity and at times some compromise to obtain the desired data.

In most situations, a physician's examination room is insufficiently treated for sources of external acoustic and electrical noise for recording evoked neurophysiological activity. To minimize the external environment as a factor, cortical AEPs should be recorded in an electrically shielded and sound isolated booth that is not adjacent to large sources of electrical or magnetic radiation such as hospital electrical distribution networks, magnetic resonance imaging (MRI) units, or mainframe computer processing centres. The power for the electrophysiological recording system and that for the stimulation system should originate from a clean source that is not compromised by periodic disruptive ground integrity checks or other sources of noise. It is important to avoid stimulus presentation rates that correspond to whole number multiples or fractions of the alternating current line frequency. For example, in North America, where 60 Hz is the line frequency, stimulation intervals of 1/s 2/s and so forth should be avoided. Use of such frequencies corresponds to a constant phase of the alternating current power source. This makes it extremely difficult to average out any contributions to the AEPs induced by line frequency noise. When non-whole number stimulation rates (for example, 1.9/s versus 2/s) are used, the phase of the power source changes for each stimulus presentation. When out of phase with the rate of stimulus presentation, induced power line noise is greatly reduced by the signal averaging process used to extract the AEPs.

Subject preparation

Another critical factor in obtaining quality AEP recordings is the procedure used to prepare the individual. Critically important is the application of EEG recording electrodes to the scalp. A common problem in electrode application is poor scalp contact for two electrodes in particular: the ground and the reference. Therefore extra effort should be made to ensure that these electrodes have particularly good contact with the scalp. This is quantified by the measured impedance between the recording electrode and the scalp, ideally below 5 kohms (at 30 Hz). In theory, the current generation of extremely high impedance recording amplifiers reduces the need for low impedance contact between electrode and scalp. However, maintaining low electrode impedances minimizes the amount of extraneous electrical activity that may be induced into the recording electrodes. As previously stated, extraneous sources of electrical activity (for example, pickup from AC power sources, radio frequency [RF] activity, and so forth) are further minimized by recording the AEPs in an electrically quiet environment such as an electrically shielded acoustic suite (also called a Faraday cage). Electrode impedances should be monitored periodically during testing to ensure that good contact with the scalp is maintained.

Recording the cortical AEPs: amplifying and filtering

Cortical AEPs are weak biological signals embedded in background EEG noise (defined as neurogenic and myogenic activity uncorrelated with the presentation of the stimulus). Therefore preamplifiers and filters are used to amplify the signals and remove unwanted noise components, or to improve the signal to noise ratio (SNR). Both the gain of the amplifiers and the passband of the filters depend on the type of AEP being recorded. Unfortunately, because of the large electrical stimulus artefact that occurs with cochlear implant stimulation, the usual filter settings for the AEPs often cannot be used. Consequently, there is heavy reliance on the process of averaging to improve the SNR.

Recording the cortical AEPs: how much data averaging is enough?

A question that is common to all AEP testing is how much averaging is sufficient to obtain a good quality recording. The answer to this depends on the amplitude of the AEPs and the amplitude of the background EEG noise. Thus, in signal processing terms, averaging should ideally continue until the amplitude of the AEP (the signal) is larger than that of the background EEG noise.

This means that the SNR should at least be greater than one. As indicated previously, cortical AEP peak-to-peak amplitudes across normally hearing subjects typically range from approximately 1 μV up to 10 μV. Peak-to-peak values in individual subjects typically range between 2 and 5 μV. Our studies indicate that the cortical AEPs recorded from CI subjects have similar amplitudes, perhaps larger in children. In contrast to this 10 μV range for AEP amplitude, the range in amplitude for background EEG noise is much larger. Figure 8.3 illustrates the magnitude of a single epoch (sweep) of background EEG recorded from one adult (upper) and one child (lower) CI user measured at electrode location Cz. For the adult, the peak-to-peak amplitude of the EEG is approximately 20 μV, excluding a large stimulus artefact that is approximately 80 μV. The background EEG for the implanted child is around 40 μV peak-to-peak: nearly twice that of the adult. Figure 8.4 shows two different

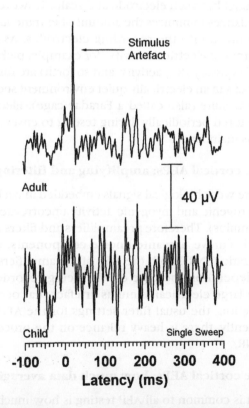

Figure 8.3. Single sweeps of EEG activity recorded from a child and adult CI user. These illustrate the differences in background EEG noise amplitude. In addition, the stimulus artefact that is clearly present in the ongoing EEG of the adult CI user, is not apparent in the EEG of the child CI user.

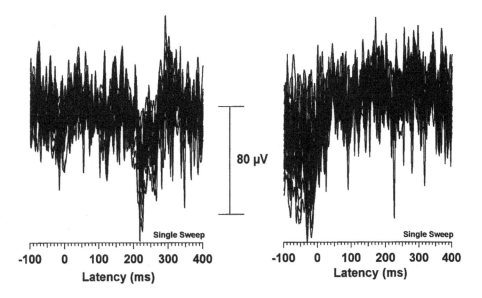

Figure 8.4. Two different single sweep epochs recorded from the same implanted child. Data from all 30 scalp electrode locations are superimposed in butterfly plots. For this individual, peak-to-peak amplitude of the background EEG ranges between 40 and 80 µV. These data highlight the changes in background EEG noise amplitude that can occur within and across recording epochs.

single sweep epochs of EEG recorded from another implanted child measured at 30 scalp electrode locations (note the absence of stimulus artefact). The data from all the scalp electrodes are superimposed in a butterfly plot. For the first 100 ms of the second single sweep, EEG peak-to-peak amplitude exceeds 80 µV, after which it reduces to a level around 60 µV peak-to-peak. The activity shown in these figures illustrates two important points. First, the amplitude of background EEG noise can vary greatly from individual to individual. Second, within an individual, the level of EEG noise may vary not only across epochs but even within recording epochs.

This variability in the cortical AEP amplitude and background EEG noise makes determination of the exact amount of data that is sufficient for AEP detection and identification more difficult. Objective, online methods of evoked potential detection have been developed for activity evoked in the auditory brainstem pathway (for example Don et al., 1984; Elberling and Don, 1984). However, these objective detection techniques require conditions of signal stationarity (minimal neurophysiological variability in the evoked activity) and a degree of background EEG noise independence from the signal. These conditions do not exist for cortical evoked activity. While there have been efforts to develop objective measures for offline detection of certain cortical AEPs (Guthrie and Buchwald, 1991; Ponton et al., 1997), none are implemented on commercially available neurophysiological recording systems. Consequently, clinical and research studies of cortical potentials typically rely on other approaches to determine how much data to collect. Subjective methods of evoked potential detection rely heavily on the ability of a trained observer to visually identify the neurophysiological response from the background EEG. Once the AEPs are identified visually, data collection stops. This approach can be very time efficient, but even 'expert' observers may incorrectly identify noise peaks that have the appropriate morphologies and latencies. The commonly used alternative to this approach is to continue data acquisition until a predetermined number of stimuli have been presented. This approach, typically used to collect AEP data in research protocols, is not particularly time efficient. Moreover, when moderate to high levels of background EEG noise are present, the amount of data collected may still be insufficient to confidently identify the AEPs.

The amount of data needed to obtain reasonable quality cortical AEPs can at least be roughly estimated by applying the basic principles of signal averaging. When the AEP is extracted by signal averaging, the amplitude of the averaged residual non-time-locked EEG noise reduces as a function of $1/\sqrt{n}$, where n is the number of sweeps. This function is illustrated in Figure 8.5. In this figure, peak-to-peak averaged residual amplitude is plotted as a function of the number of averaged sweeps. Note that the number of sweeps shown on the x-axis is plotted on a logarithmic scale. Five curves are plotted on this graph to represent the averaged residual amplitude of the background EEG noise after averaging for different numbers of sweeps. The labels on these curves represent set background EEG noise levels from very low (10.0 μV) to moderately high (100 μV) that cover the range for the data shown in Figures 8.3 and 8.4, and the levels commonly encountered. For these theoretical functions, the level of background noise is assumed to be constant during the AEP recordings. As shown in these graphs, the signal averaging process results in a non-linear reduction in averaged residual background noise. The largest decreases occur in the initial stages of averaging and smaller changes occur in later stages. For this illustration, we have assumed that the peak-to-peak amplitude of the AEP is approximately 5 μV (in the moderately high amplitude range for normally hearing subjects).

It is clear from Figure 8.5 that the number of sweeps required to produce AEPs with a SNR of 1 (amplitude of AEP equals that of the background noise) varies greatly as a function of the background EEG noise level. If the subject is extremely quiet (single sweep background noise ≤ 25 μV), as few as 20 to 30 averaged sweeps may be required to produce AEPs with a SNR of 1. Under these background noise conditions, at least 100 averaged sweeps are

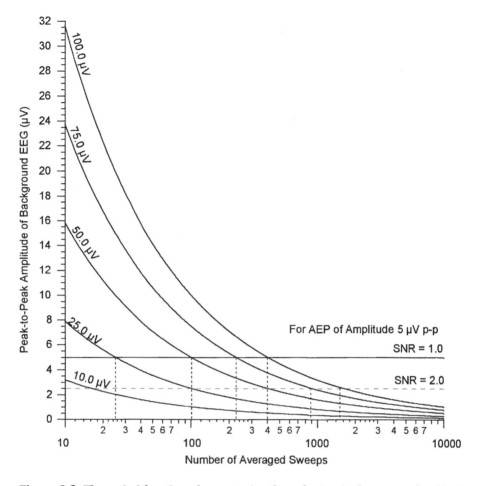

Figure 8.5. Theoretical functions demonstrating the reduction in the averaged residual background EEG noise as a function of signal averaging. Functions are shown for five background noise levels (assumed to remain constant during the period of data collection). Two horizontal SNR functions (SNR = 1 and SNR = 2) are plotted for an AEP with a peak-to-peak amplitude of 5 μV.

required to generate AEPs with a SNR of 2. It has been our experience that such low levels of background EEG are very unusual in normally hearing subjects and extremely unusual in patient populations such as CI users who may be anxious about the testing. More typical single-sweep levels of background EEG noise are represented by the functions for 25 μV through 75 μV. An EEG noise level of 50 μV requires at least 100 averaged sweeps to obtain AEPs with a SNR of 1 and more than 400 averaged sweeps to increase the SNR to a value of 2. If the noise level rises to a moderately high value of

75 µV, approximately 250 averaged sweeps are necessary to generate a SNR of 1, and more than 800 averaged sweeps to obtain a SNR of 2.

Several important points are illustrated by Figure 8.5. First, if the AEPs are smaller than expected (in this example, less than 5 µV), more sweeps (and more data collection time) are required to record AEPs of a specified SNR. Second, taking steps to minimize the background EEG noise reduces test time and/or generates higher quality (larger SNR) AEPs. In practical terms, background noise levels can be reduced by ensuring that there is good recording electrode contact with the scalp and that the subject is made as comfortable as possible. Third, only if the subject is very quiet (extremely low background EEG noise) and the AEPs are large in amplitude (>5 µV), is it possible to obtain minimal quality (SNR $\geq$ 1) responses in less than 100 sweeps. Based on the background noise levels we have observed across several hundred recording sessions of both normally hearing and implant subjects, at least 100 to 200 sweeps are necessary to generate AEPs with SNRs approaching a value of 1. AEPs based on fewer than 100 to 200 single sweeps must be considered and interpreted with much caution. Unfortunately, many published studies report AEPs that are based only on 100 or 200 averaged sweeps. Obtaining better quality AEPs with a SNR $\geq$ 2 requires more averaging, perhaps as many as 400 to 800 sweeps. At a stimulus presentation rate of approximately 1.9/second, the testing time required to obtain a single average based on 400 to 800 sweeps is approximately four to eight minutes. The drawback to spending more time collecting data for a single stimulus condition is that fewer conditions can be included in a test protocol. However, the AEPs generated by averaging larger numbers of sweeps should be more reliable, and more easily interpretable.

Selection of stimulus and stimulus artefact

Ideally, the selection of stimuli used to elicit the cortical AEPs should be based simply on the topic of interest. For example, examination of speech-related cortical activity in the AEPs should be elicited using speech sounds. However, with CI users, the electrical artefact generated by the implant hardware must be considered when selecting stimuli. Virtually all of the laboratories that record cortical AEPs from CI populations frequently encounter stimulus artefacts that are many times larger in magnitude than the AEP itself. As shown in Figures 8.1 and 8.3, the stimulus artefact is often clearly visible even in a single epoch of the ongoing EEG. Figure 8.6 contains cortical AEPs recorded from 30 scalp electrode locations showing the stimulus artefact generated by a series of 10 closely spaced (2 ms stimulus onset to onset) 100 µs voltage pulses (total duration 18.1 ms). While this CI user was fitted with the Nucleus CI22M cochlear implant, the stimulus artefact problem exists for all the implant makes that we have tested. In

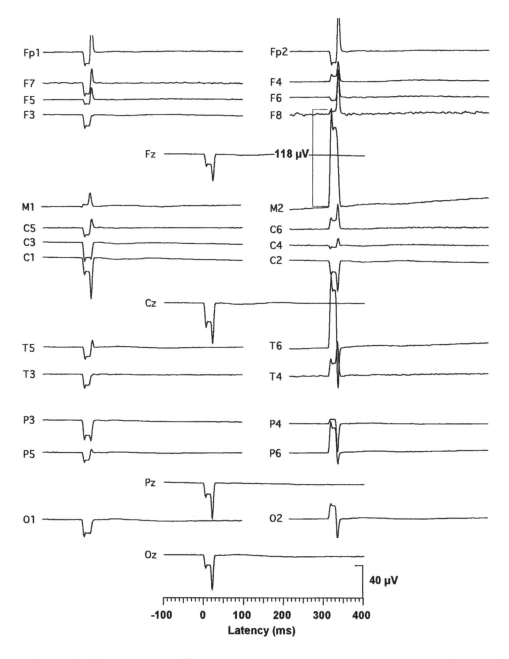

Figure 8.6. Set of cortical AEPs recorded at 30 scalp electrode locations, plotted at a y-axis scale that highlights the full excursion of the stimulus artefact. The amplitude of the stimulus artefact varies as a function of proximity to the implant, located on the right side of the head.

Figure 8.6, the y-axis scale is set to the maximum peak-to-peak amplitude of the stimulus artefact (118 µV) recorded at the right mastoid (electrode M2). At this scale setting, the cortical AEPs are not visible in the averaged responses. It is also evident from Figure 8.6 that the amplitude of the artefact varies as a function of scalp location. Compared with the amplitude of the stimulus artefact recorded at electrode M2 (118 µV), the amplitude of the artefact measured on the same side of the head at electrode C4 is 12.7 µV peak-to-peak. This is further illustrated in Figure 8.7. On the left side of this figure, the cortical AEPs recorded at Cz and C4 are scaled so that the amplitude of the stimulus artefact is the same at both electrode locations. On the right side, the AEPs recorded at electrodes C4 and Cz are shown at the same amplitude scale, which highlights the AEPs. In absolute terms, the peak-to-peak amplitudes of the AEPs recorded at Cz and C4 are actually quite similar, while the magnitude of the stimulus artefact differs by a factor of five. Due to individual differences in the geometry of the implant hardware relative to the array of recording electrodes placed on the scalp, the amplitude and polarity of the stimulus artefact varies across individuals.

Clearly, stimulus artefact poses a serious problem when recording cortical AEPs from CI users. The stimulus artefact is not apparent in the AEPs of all implanted subjects. This is illustrated by the single sweep data shown in Figure 8.4. Moreover, the artefact, when present, varies in magnitude as a function of scalp location, as shown in Figures 8.6 and 8.7. It can also vary across test sessions for a single individual. Thus far, factors that predict which CI users (including which implant type) are more likely to produce cortical AEPs containing a large stimulus artefact have not been identified. For the purposes of AEP applications, much would be gained by a thorough investigation of these factors and what could be done to eliminate this artefact. Until these factors are identified, alternative strategies must be employed that reliably isolate the stimulus artefact from the epoch containing the AEPs of interest. For example, one very successful strategy employed at the House Ear Institute is to simply limit stimuli to very short durations, typically less than 40 ms. The AEPs shown in Figures 8.6 and 8.7 are examples of this approach. These AEPs were recorded using biphasic current pulses (200 µs/phase) presented in short duration trains to drive the implant. A relatively high sampling rate (for cortical AEPs) of 1,000 Hz was chosen to record the incoming EEG. This allowed the use of wide passband settings (maximum allowed) for the input filters on the EEG amplifiers. Although the artefact is clearly present in the AEPs, and is much larger in magnitude than any neural activity, it is sufficiently contained and isolated in the early portion of the recording epoch so that the later cortical AEPs are undistorted and clearly represented. For almost all CI users tested thus far, these recording conditions (short stimulus durations, wide-filter passbands) have been sufficient

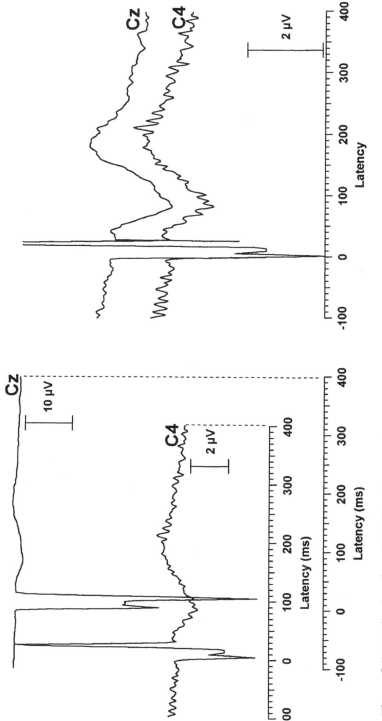

Figure 8.7. Amplitudes of cortical AEPs relative to the stimulus artefact. On the right, the variation in stimulus artefact amplitude as a function of nearby scalp locations is highlighted. On the left, the size of the AEPs is compared for the same nearby pair of electrodes.

to prevent the stimulus artefact from smearing extensively into the response epoch containing the AEPs of interest. If a very narrow filter passband were used on the input stages of the EEG amplifiers (for example 1 to 30 Hz), it is likely that the stimulus artefact would be smeared across at least part of the epoch containing the AEPs.

Use of a short stimulus that isolates the artefact from the AEP epoch of interest is not possible when using speech segments. At best, a speech segment might be reduced in length to 50 to 75 ms. However, reducing the duration can affect intelligibility. It also precludes the use of full words as stimuli. Ponton et al. are currently evaluating an advanced signal processing approach to this problem based on a technique described by Jutten and Herault (1991), Bell and Sejnowski (1995) and Makeig et al. (1996; 1997, and 1999a,b) to remove blink artefacts from EEG data. The technique, independent components analysis (ICA), is similar to principle components analysis (PCA). In contrast to PCA, which attempts to separate or decorrelate data into orthogonal components, ICA attempts to represent the EEG or AEP signal as a set of statistically independent components (Hyvärinen and Oja, 2000). While PCA models the data into orthogonal components that have minimal first order correlations, ICA models the data as components in which second order and higher order correlations are near zero. Unlike PCA, ICA generates components that tend to be more physiologically plausible. An illustration of this technique for the removal of stimulus artefact is shown in Figure 8.8.

Figure 8.8a (upper) contains a butterfly plot (waveforms from all electrodes superimposed with a bandpass of 0 to 200 Hz) of the cortical AEPs recorded from an adult CI user. The AEP waveforms are dominated by a large stimulus artefact generated by words presented through the speech processor of a Nucleus CI22M device. The stimulus artefact varies in amplitude across electrode locations but persists for the 500 ms duration of the word. The mean global field power (MGFP) is shown below the butterfly plot. The MGFP provides a measure (standard deviation) of the instantaneous activity at each time point for the evoked potentials measured at all scalp locations. This representation of the cortical AEPs clearly shows the domination of the stimulus artefact. Dipole modelling of this activity across the normal latency range of the P1–N1–P2 interval (50 to 250 ms) identified a source located on the lower right side of the head model posterior to the ear, between the outer two shells (skull and skin), appropriate for the location of the implant hardware. When these data were subjected to ICA, as shown in Figure 8.8b (lowest) four major components were apparent. The first component, shown at the top of the figure, represents the stimulus artefact. This component has a loading factor more than six times larger than the next component (5.92 versus 0.93), which most likely represents part of the

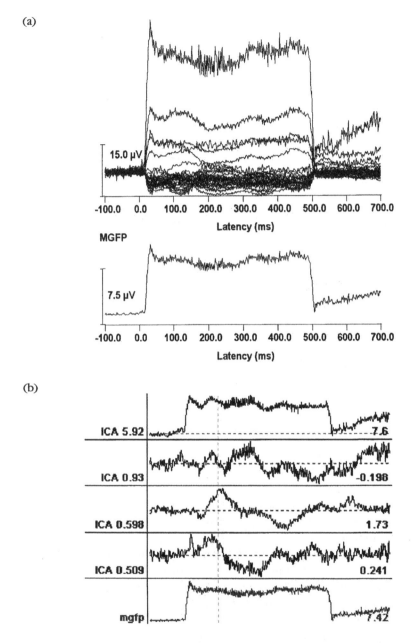

Figure 8.8. Demonstration of independent components analysis for the removal of stimulus artefact. (a) Upper: a butterfly plot with the cortical AEPs superimposed for all electrode locations. Lower: the mean global field power (MGFP). Both representations of the cortical AEPs are dominated by a large response representing the stimulus artefact. (b) Lowest ICA results showing four major loadings. The largest represents the stimulus artefact, while the other components represent neural activity.

evoked neural response. The effects of extracting this component are shown in Figure 8.8c. Both the butterfly plot and the MGFP contain clear peaks corresponding in latency to the N1 and P2 peaks of the cortical AEP. Figure 8.8d contrasts individual AEP waveforms prior to and after ICA extraction of the stimulus artefact. These waveforms have also been subjected to zero-phase low-pass filtering at 30 Hz (12 dB/octave). The activity at electrode site C3, contralateral to the implant remains essentially the same prior to and after the ICA extraction process. However, there was a significant reduction of artefact contamination at electrode C4, ipsilateral to the implant. This reduction is even more evident at electrode P6, located close to the implant hardware. Source modelling of the AEPs following extraction of the stimulus artefact generated a solution with symmetrically positioned dipoles located in the auditory cortex of the left and right hemispheres.

As this example illustrates, ICA provides a method by which stimulus artefact may be isolated and extracted from the AEPs. This method is particularly useful when the artefact of stimuli such as word segments or full words has a duration that overlaps the AEP epoch of interest. However, successful application of this technique requires that the number of electrodes exceeds the number of meaningful ICA components within the data. Typically, the cortical AEP is characterized by three to five ICA components. An initial analysis suggests that at least eight to ten electrodes are required to adequately characterize and isolate the artefact for a full extraction.

Recording the mismatch negativity

As a passively recorded, neurophysiological correlate of auditory discrimination, the MMN has the potential to be a powerful technique for assessing auditory short-term memory and discrimination processes that may be important prerequisites for spoken language processing. The drawback of the MMN is that the time required to record this AEP can be considerable. Moreover, attempts to shorten the data collection may make interpretation difficult, if not impossible.

The basic methodology for recording the MMN is quite simple. An oddball sequence is used containing one frequently repeated stimulus, randomly interspersed with one or more infrequently presented physically deviant stimuli. The MMN represents an added negative component contained in the AEPs evoked by the presentation of the deviant stimulus. The oddball sequence is typically pseudorandom, with the condition that two deviants should not occur sequentially. According to Ritter et al. (1995) a condition of at least two consecutively presented standards is required to establish the memory trace that triggers the neural generators producing the MMN. In most published studies, the frequency of occurrence for the deviant stimulus ranges between 10 and 20%.

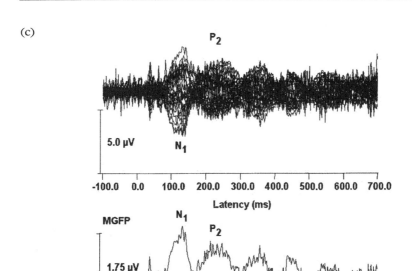

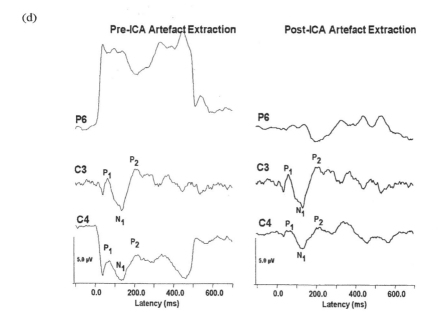

Figure 8.8. (c) Following extraction of the artefact component, peaks are present in both the butterfly plot and MGFP corresponding in latency to the N1 and P2 peaks of the cortical AEP. (d) The effects of the ICA extraction are illustrated for AEPs at individual electrodes positioned at scalp locations contralateral (C3) and ipsilateral (C4 and P6) to the implant hardware.

In studies of normally hearing populations, many physical (acoustic) differences have been used to evoked the MMN, including basic psychoacoustic contrasts such as frequency, duration, and intensity. These contrasts have been used in isolation and in combination with each other. Other more complex stimulus differences have also been used, including consonant-vowel (CV) contrasts based on voice onset time, formant frequency, and formant frequency transition duration. Kraus et al. (1993) have also used CV syllable contrasts to evoke the MMN in CI users. Initially, the MMN was considered to simply reflect a sensitivity to differences in the acoustical properties of stimuli. This conclusion was based on studies of the MMN evoked by CV syllable contrasts taken from a continuum of synthetically generated speech sounds (for example, Sharma et al., 1993). Results of these studies showed that the magnitude of the MMN evoked by speech sounds within a phonetic category was the same size as that evoked by stimuli crossing the categorical boundary. These findings suggested that the MMN reflects the processing of the acoustics of the speech stimulus, but not phonetic processing into categories. However, recent studies have shown that the MMN may also reflect cortical processes underlying phonetic categories changes (Dehaene-Lambertz, 1997; Näätänen et al., 1997; Cheour et al., 1998), including coding of native versus non-native language contrasts (Winkler et al., 1999; Sharma and Dorman, 2000; Näätänen, 2001).

The standard method for derivation and presentation of the MMN is to subtract the response evoked by the standard stimulus from that evoked by the deviant stimulus, producing a difference waveform. However, two divergent derivation approaches exist, which are distinguished based on the response used as the standard stimulus. The data shown in Figure 8.9, representing the AEPs evoked by a /ba/ – /da/ speech segment contrast in a normally hearing subject highlight these divergent approaches. Figure 8.9a illustrates one commonly used approach. This figure shows the AEPs evoked by /da/ as the standard superimposed on the AEP evoked by the deviant stimulus /ba/. The derived difference waveform (shown below) contains a component that appears MMN-like in polarity, magnitude and latency. As stated previously, the MMN is defined as an added negative component in the AEPs evoked by the occurrence of a *deviant* stimulus. Therefore, it is the context of deviance that evokes the MMN. Implicit to this definition is the assumption that the obligatory potentials for the /ba/ and /da/ syllables generate equivalent (or nearly so) obligatory AEPs when presented as the standard stimulus or in isolation (equivalent to the deviant-alone condition described by, for example, Kraus and McGee, 1993; Kraus et al., 1993). Figure 8.9b contains the AEPs evoked by the /ba/ and /da/ syllables when presented as standards. Clearly, in this example the assumption of equivalent standard AEPs is violated. A difference waveform

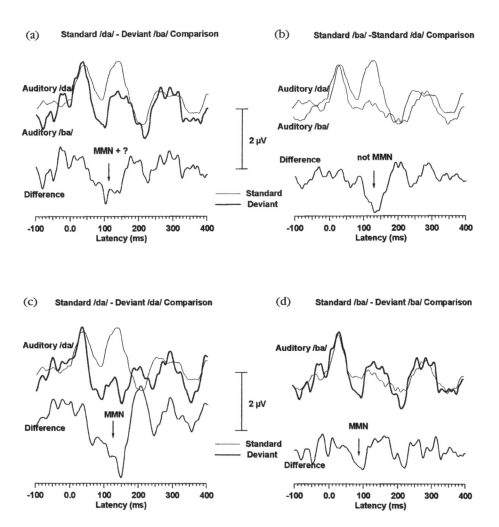

Figure 8.9. Methods of MMN derivation. (a) represents the commonly used method of subtracting the response of the standard AEP from that of the deviant AEP. This derivation does not control for possible differences in the obligatory AEPs evoked by each stimulus when presented as the standard in isolation as shown in (b) which contains AEPs for /ba/ and /da/ as the standard with the resulting difference waveform shown below. Figures (c) and (d) contain derivations of the MMN that control for physical differences in the obligatory AEPs by holding the stimulus constant and changing the context in which it is presented.

is also shown, produced by subtracting the AEPs evoked by the standard /da/ from those evoked by the standard /ba/. The result is a difference waveform that contains activity that is MMN-like in latency, amplitude and morphology. However, the activity represented in the difference waveform does not fulfil the definition of the MMN. Evidence of these large differences in the obligatory AEPs for /ba/ and /da/ violates this critical assumption underlying the derivation of the MMN. Therefore, interpreting the nature of the activity contained in the difference waveform of Figure 8.9a is at least made more complicated, and perhaps completely confounded. This waveform may contain MMN activity. It may contain components of the MMN plus differences in the obligatory AEPs. However, it may simply represent the differences in the obligatory AEPs of the /ba/ and /da/ stimuli.

An alternative derivation of the MMN that controls for possible differences in the obligatory potentials is the inclusion of a deviant-alone condition, most consistently employed by Kraus and colleagues (for example Kraus and McGee, 1993; Kraus et al., 1993). Using the /ba/ – /da/ contrast as an example, two presentation sequences are required to derive the MMN. One sequence is the standard oddball task, with the infrequently presented deviant /ba/ stimulus embedded in a sequence of frequently presented /da/ stimuli. In the other sequence, the AEPs evoked by the deviant /ba/ presented in isolation are recorded. The MMN is derived by subtracting the AEPs evoked by deviant-alone /ba/ from those evoked by the deviant /ba/ in the oddball condition. This derivation provides the necessary control for possible differences in the obligatory AEPs evoked by the standard and deviant stimuli. Consequently, the activity contained in the difference waveform should represent the uncontaminated effects of the context change from standard to deviant.

Figures 8.9c and 8.9d illustrate a variation on the deviant-alone approach that we have used in our studies of the MMN in normally hearing and cochlear implant populations. In this approach, two oddball sequences are recorded. In one sequence, the /da/ is presented as the standard and the /ba/ is presented as the deviant. In the other sequence, the context of the standard and the deviant are reversed, so that the /da/ is presented as the deviant and the /ba/ is presented as the standard. This results in two sets of MMN data, one in which /da/ as the standard is contrasted with /da/ presented as the deviant (Figure 8.9c), and a second with a /ba/ standard, /ba/ deviant contrast. Like the deviant-alone condition, this approach also controls for possible differences in the obligatory AEPs of the two contrasted stimuli. In Figure 8.9c, the difference waveform contains a large negativity peaking in amplitude at about 150 ms. The /ba/ contrast shown in Figure 8.9d also shows evidence of a negativity, although smaller in amplitude and earlier in latency than that observed for the standard-deviant /da/ contrast. These apparent amplitude and latency asymmetries are common (the /da/ MMN appearing very different from the /ba/ MMN). We have observed these asymmetries with other stimulus contrasts (Ponton and Don, 1995). Although a clear reason for this asymmetry is not apparent, there may be parallels in studies of speech recognition that show perceptual order effects (for example, Mann and Soli, 1991).

In summary, use of the MMN as a preperceptual measure of auditory short-term memory discrimination processes is well established. However, it is important to maintain an appropriate methodology to record this AEP. It has been suggested that the method for deriving the MMN described in Figure 8.9a is sufficient and that any differences in the AEPs evoked by non-physically identical standards and deviants is evidence, at some level, that the cortex is making a distinction between the two stimuli. This is a valid point. However, two distinct cortical networks may be involved in these processes. One network may be differentially sensitive to the acoustic features of a stimulus without invoking any process that correlates with perceptual discrimination. This, by definition, would not be the mismatch negativity as it is not dependent on the development of a memory trace and does not require the oddball presentation sequence to register differences. Nevertheless, this sensitivity of the obligatory AEPs to differences in speech sounds can be exploited to further understand the relationship between auditory system activation and spoken language perception. On the other hand, the cortical network underlying the MMN is presumably a comparator process that compares the memory representation of the standard with that of the infrequently presented deviant. When this comparator network is activated by a difference between the standard and the deviant stimuli, an additional component is generated in response to the deviant, producing the MMN.

Objective detection of the mismatch negativity

If good quality cortical AEP data have been acquired (high number of averaged sweeps and low background noise), the obligatory peaks can be easily identified, allowing the measurement of latencies and amplitudes for each. Detection of the MMN can be much more difficult. Like the cortical AEPs, the MMN is often identified subjectively, based on visual detection. As mentioned previously, visual detection of the obligatory cortical AEPs even by expert observers can be erroneous. The potential for inaccurate identification is even greater for the MMN for several reasons. First, the obligatory cortical AEPs are usually identified from a response containing a relatively larger number of averaged sweeps to obtain an acceptable SNR (either explicitly or implicitly). In research applications, we have used anywhere from 400 to 2,000 sweeps to generate the final averaged response. Since the MMN is contained in the waveform evoked by an *infrequently* presented deviant stimulus, the averaged deviant response is based on a much smaller number of averaged sweeps, with a consequently poorer SNR. For example, if a total of 500 stimulus presentations are used to evoke the MMN, and the occurrence of the deviant is 15% (about average for MMN studies), only 75 sweeps are contained in the averaged response to the deviant stimulus. As previously described (and shown in Figure 8.5), the SNR for AEPs containing only 75 averaged sweeps is likely to be poor (SNR <1). If 1,000 stimulus presentations are used to evoke the MMN, the deviant AEPs will be based on only 150 averaged sweeps. While the amplitude of the MMN can be quite large (> 2 µV), it is typically smaller than the AEPs evoked by the standards and deviants used in the oddball task. Moreover, the SNR of the MMN is further degraded by the subtraction process used to derive the difference waveform. Clearly, recording the MMN with an acceptable SNR (SNR ≥ 1) requires a significant investment in data collection time.

With these unavoidable decrements in the SNR of the waveform containing the MMN, an objective method for detecting this response is preferred. Two statistical approaches have been used. One approach has employed point-by-point, pairwise comparisons between groups of standard and deviant AEPs across subjects using t-tests. Appropriate adjustments for using multiple t-tests and for correlations between adjacent data points are applied to determine whether the MMN is present in the data set. This objective technique is clearly an improvement over subjective detection of the MMN. Unfortunately, it requires low noise conditions that typically only exist in group data, making it unsuitable for the purpose of MMN detection in the single subject.

We have developed an alternative statistic, described in Ponton et al. (1997), that is specifically structured for detection of the MMN in individual subjects. The basic assumption underlying this statistic is that the MMN represents an added negative component in the evoked response to the deviant stimulus. Figure 8.10 summarizes the steps in generating the statistic. To detect the added negative component representing the MMN, the scalp-recorded waveforms (Figure 8.10a) are transformed into low noise waveforms (both standard and deviant) by mathematically integrating the AEPs (Figure 8.10b). This integration is simply the recalculation of each data point in the waveform as a cumulative sum. Next, an estimate of the variability in the integrated AEP waveforms evoked by the standard stimulus is generated. In our data collection protocol, presentation sequences typically consist of about 2,200 sweeps, approximately 200 to 250 of these containing activity evoked by the deviant. To obtain an estimate of variability in the AEPs evoked by the standard stimulus, the 1,900 to 2,000 sweeps containing activity evoked by the standard stimulus are randomly sampled to generate a set of subaverages. For this purpose, a randomization (Edgington, 1995) or Monte Carlo approach is employed to generate a set of 200 subaverages. Thus, each subaverage contains approximately 200 randomly selected sweeps evoked by the standard stimulus (the number 200 being approximately equal to the number of averaged sweeps comprising the deviant AEP

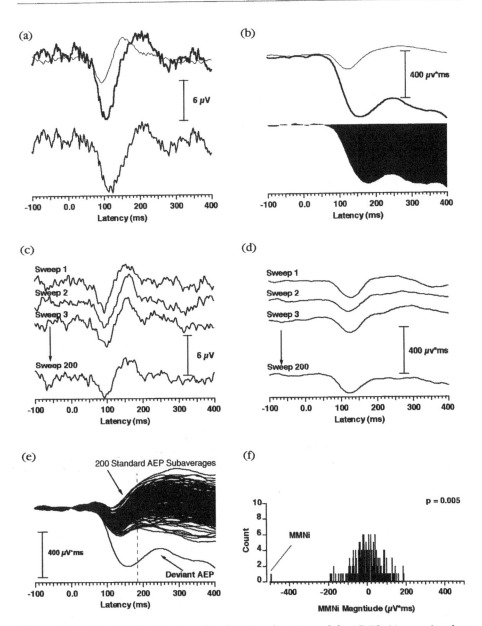

Figure 8.10. The MMNi technique for objective detection of the MMN. (a) contains the superimposed standard and deviant AEPs (thin and thick lines respectively) with the difference waveform shown below. (b) contains the integrated AEPs with the difference waveform plotted as a solid area. (c) contains the AEP subaverages used to generate a distribution of the standard AEP variability. (d) contains integrated derivations of the standard AEP subaverages shown in (c). (e) the integrated deviant AEP is superimposed on the set of 200 standard AEP subaverages. The dashed vertical line marks the latency value selected a priori for comparing magnitude of the deviant AEP and the standard AEP subaverages. (f) contains the distribution of MMNi magnitudes for the standard and deviant AEPs. An exact probability value is also shown.

waveform). Each of these standard response subaverages is then integrated. This is shown in Figures 8.10c and 8.10d. Then, at a fixed, a priori-selected latency, the magnitude of the integrated deviant AEP is compared to that of the distribution formed by the 200 standard AEP subaverages (Figures 8.10e and 8.10f) and an exact probability value is obtained. The result is a distribution-free statistic that is entirely self-contained, and constructed specifically to detect the MMN in the individual subject.

To illustrate the principles of the integrated MMN (MMNi) technique, data from an easy-to-discriminate stimulus contrast was used for the example shown in Figure 8.10. This contrast was based on a difference in the duration of two current pulse click trains. Each click train consisted of a series of biphasic current pulses with the onset of each pulse separated by a 2 ms interval. The MMN illustrated in Figure 8.10 was evoked by a 12 ms duration difference, produced by contrasting trains of 10 pulses (18 ms in duration) and 4 pulses (6 ms in duration) in length. The MMN represents the difference between AEPs evoked by a 10-click train presented as the standard compared to the AEPs evoked by the same stimulus presented as the deviant. Figure 8.11 contains (from left to right) the 12 ms contrast shown in Figure 8.10, as well as shorter duration contrasts of 8 ms and 4 ms. Scalp-recorded AEPs evoked by the standard and deviant stimuli (thin and thick lines, respectively) are shown for each contrast at the top of the figure, with the corresponding integrated standard and deviant responses shown below. The solid areas represent the integrated difference waveforms for each condition. These responses are plotted as a solid, since, by definition, the integrated response represents an area (cumulative amplitude as a function of duration). Distributions of standard AEP subaverages with exact probability values are shown at the bottom for each of the contrasts. This example shows that as the duration difference becomes smaller, there is a reduction in the magnitude of the MMNi, most notable between the 12 ms and 8 ms duration difference conditions. There is a corresponding change in probability from a very significant difference ($p = 0.005$ indicating a large magnitude MMN) to a smaller value bordering significance ($p = 0.060$ and $p = 0.045$) for the two shorter duration contrasts. Behaviourally, this individual was able to distinguish the 12 ms duration difference in the click trains with 100% accuracy. Performance dropped to 86% for the 8 ms duration contrast and below threshold, to 66% for the 4 ms duration contrast. This single-subject analysis demonstrates a moderate correspondence between the behaviourally determined discrimination threshold and the neurophysiologically determined MMN threshold.

The data shown in Figure 8.11 were taken from a study assessing click train duration discrimination in normally hearing and CI adults. Behavioural threshold was defined as 75% correct on a two alternative forced choice task

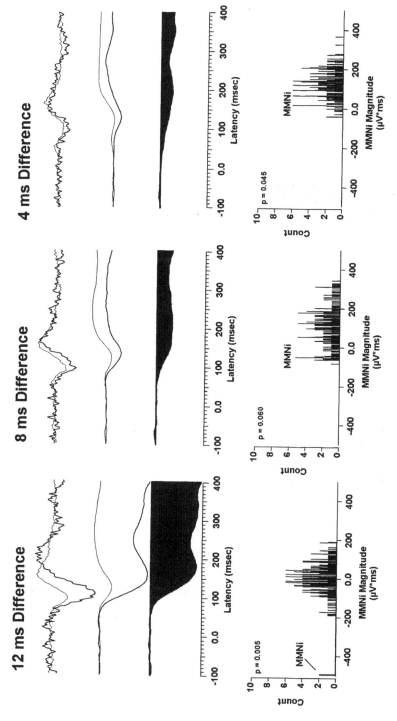

Figure 8.11. Series of duration contrasts demonstrating the reduction in magnitude of MMN as the duration difference decreases. Time waveforms, integrated responses, magnitude distributions, and exact probability values are shown for each contrast.

(same/different response) and neurophysiological threshold was defined as p<0.01 probability of a response. The results of this study showed that all normally hearing subjects had better behaviourally determined than neuro-physiologically determined (MMN) discrimination thresholds for these duration contrasts. With the exception of one individual, the opposite result was obtained for CI adults; neurophysiologically determined thresholds were lower than behavioural thresholds. Perhaps the most notable finding in this study was that overall, the neurophysiologically determined threshold based on the MMN was the same (no significant difference) for normally hearing and CI subjects (Trautwein et al., 1998).

Review of cortical AEP studies with CI users

The application of cortical AEPs in CI users has a very short history. The first cortical recording of AEPs from CI users was reported by Pelizzone, Hari and colleagues (Pelizzone et al., 1986, 1987, 1991; Hari et al., 1988). These studies demonstrated that the obligatory components of the cortical-evoked activity could be reliably recorded from adult CI users, and that these responses were fundamentally similar to those obtained from normally hearing adults. Kraus et al. (1993) completed the first systematic analysis of speech-evoked MMN activity in CI users using a voice onset time /pa/–/ba/ contrast. Results showed that as a group, individuals with good CI-assisted speech perception had much more robust MMNs than those CI users who showed only marginal benefit in speech recognition. In contrast, the cortical AEPs recorded from those individuals with poor speech perception showed little evidence of a MMN in the difference waveforms.

Our cortical AEP research with CI users has not used speech segments (due to stimulus artefact problems). We have focused on issues of cortical processing that ultimately increase our understanding of the variability in spoken language processing skills found in CI subjects. These studies have included investigations of possible differences in the origins of cortical activity between normally hearing and CI adults. We have also extensively investigated the effects of deafness and cochlear implant use on the matura-tion of the central nervous system. The results of these studies have led to more recent attempts to use neurophysiological responses as measures for constructing and monitoring training programmes for CI users. The prelimi-nary results of the training studies suggest that cortical AEPs may have an important clinical function when working with adults and children who use a cochlear implant. Finally, it is important to note that all of the work described in the following section was completed with the use of special computerized hardware (Shannon et al., 1990) that provides direct control over activation of the Nucleus CI22M cochlear implant.

Localization of auditory activity in the CI user

Studies of cortical plasticity have suggested that the functional organization of the cortex is not fixed. Rather, functional organization may change dramatically as a result of absence of normal sensory input (for example, McCandlish et al., 1996). Individuals who are fitted with a cochlear implant experience a period of auditory deprivation due to profound deafness, a period that may vary considerably across individuals. Therefore, we investigated whether the absence of input and the reintroduction of auditory stimulation with a CI might change the localization of auditory cortical activity in CI users (Ponton et al., 1993 and 2000a). Localization of the evoked auditory activity in normally hearing and CI subjects was based on dipole source modelling (see Scherg, 1990 for a review of source modelling theory) and focused specifically on the N1-P2 activity in the obligatory cortical AEPs. Results of this analysis showed that the source location of cortical AEPs was similar for normally hearing adults and CI users who had normal hearing until adulthood and then subsequently became deaf. The AEPs recorded from both groups of adults produced similar source models, consistent with activation of the superior surface of the temporal lobe. The obligatory P1-N1-P2 potentials were clearly represented in tangentially oriented dipoles in each hemisphere of the modelled brain. The T-complex peaks Ta and Tb were represented in radially oriented dipole sources located in each hemisphere. The radial orientation of this source activity is considered to reflect activation of the lateral surface of the temporal lobe, presumably reflecting generators located in secondary auditory cortical areas (Scherg and von Cramon, 1986). Ponton et al. (1993) also included some provocative source modelling results from one implanted child. Like the adults tested in this study, the AEPs recorded from this CI child localized to the superior temporal lobe in the head model. Moreover, an apparent cochleotopic change in source location was also observed. As stimulation changed from more basal to more apical cochlear positions, the source location moved from a more posterior to anterior position in the head model. Unfortunately, this result has been hard to replicate in other CI users, perhaps reflecting the complex representation of tonotopic maps in primary cortical areas (Kaas and Hacket, 2000). In other analyses, we assessed source localization of the MMN in normally hearing and implanted adults (Ponton et al., 2000b). Like the findings for the obligatory cortical AEPs, source locations for the MMN were consistent with superior temporal cortex activation (the MMN is represented in tangentially oriented dipoles for both subject groups).

Effects of age of onset/period of deafness on cortical AEP morphology

Figure 8.12 contains representative cortical AEPs recorded from the scalp electrode Cz from CI users, and the grand mean waveforms recorded at the same scalp location for normally hearing adults and children. The AEPs of the adult CI users were recorded from individuals who had normal hearing until adulthood and then became profoundly deaf for a period of time prior to being implanted. As mentioned previously, the cortical AEPs of adult CI users with late-onset deafness are similar to those of normally hearing adults. Latencies of the AEP peaks P1 and N1 are very similar in both groups (lower traces). The latency of the P2 peak appears to be somewhat prolonged in latency compared with that of normally hearing subjects, but this may be

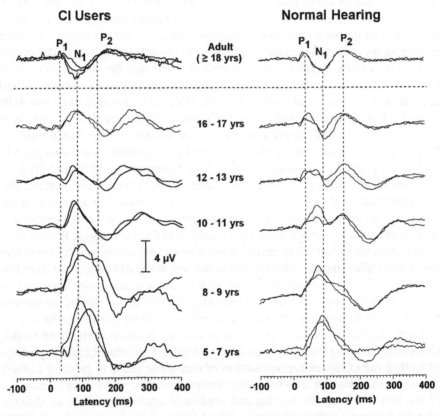

Figure 8.12. AEPs recorded from cochlear implant users and normally hearing subjects. The cortical AEPs from the normally hearing subjects represent grand mean waveforms. For CI users, the AEPs are from representative individual subjects. The adult CI users had hearing as children and became profoundly deaf as adults. The AEPs of both normally hearing and CI younger children (5–9 years of age) are dominated by a large positivity (labelled P1). The AEPs of the normally hearing children show the emergence of the N1 peak at 10–11 years of age. Although there is a reduction in AEP amplitude for the CI children and some latency change, the morphology stays essentially unchanged (i.e. no emergence of N1).

related to an age difference between the groups. Most of the cortical AEPs for normally hearing adults shown in Figure 8.12 were obtained from individuals between 18 and 20 years of age. In contrast the AEPs of the adult CI users came from individuals who were all older than 25 years of age.

While the cortical AEPs of normally hearing and implanted adults are generally similar, distinct differences in the AEPs of normally hearing and implanted children emerge during adolescence. In five-to-seven-year-olds, cortical AEP morphology is quite similar for normally hearing and implanted children. The AEPs are dominated by a large positivity with a peak latency around 100 ms. However, by 10 to 11 years of age, morphologies of the cortical AEPs for normally hearing and implanted children begin to diverge. In normally hearing children, the large positivity observed at younger ages divides into two smaller positive peaks (P1 and P2, respectively) separated by a shallow negativity (N1). For the normally hearing children, age-related changes occur: P1 peak amplitude decreases, with the N1 and P2 peaks becoming the more dominant features of the AEP morphology. In contrast, the large positivity that dominates the cortical AEPs of the five-to-seven-year-old implanted children persists, although becoming somewhat shorter in latency. This positive peak, which we have labelled as P1, is followed by a negativity that has a much longer latency than the N1 measured in the cortical AEPs of normally hearing children.

We have studied extensively the maturational changes of the large positivity that dominates the AEPs of implanted children, compared to the pattern of AEP maturation in normally hearing children (Ponton et al., 1996a,b, 1999 and 2000a; Ponton and Eggermont, 2001). Our initial analyses of the age-related changes in the latency of this peak revealed a number of interesting properties (Ponton et al., 1996a,b). In implanted children, the latency of P1 was prolonged compared with that of normally hearing children. The extent to which P1 latency was prolonged correlated with the duration of deafness prior to implantation. Thus, children with a longer interval of deafness prior to implantation had more prolonged P1 latencies, with a nearly one-to-one correspondence between the duration of deafness and the extent of delayed P1 latency. This finding suggested that during the period of deafness, the cortical generators reflected in the P1 did not mature. However, P1 latency did show an apparent age-related decrease both in cross-sectional data and in longitudinal data recorded from individual implanted children. Moreover, the rate of latency change for this peak was nearly identical to the rate of P1 latency change observed in normally hearing children. Therefore, when the age of the implanted children was adjusted to account for the period of deafness prior to implantation (time-in-sound or hearing age), patterns of P1 latency maturation for the implanted and normally hearing children were indistinguishable (Ponton et al., 1996a).

The results of this study led to two conclusions. First, at least some aspects of cortical maturation require sensory input to proceed. Second, activation of the central auditory pathways by the cochlear implant appears sufficient to restore normal rates of cortical maturation for at least some cortical processes. It was therefore concluded that given enough time, and the absence of a restricted time period for maturation, the cortical AEPs of CI children would ultimately become indistinguishable from their normally hearing peers.

The cortical AEP data reported in the previous study included CI children up to 12 to 13 years of age. A subsequent longitudinal follow-up of several of the CI children revealed an unexpected finding (Ponton et al., 1999; Ponton and Eggermont, 2001). After about 12 years of age, maturational changes in the latency of the P1 AEP no longer occurred. Thus, as these children progressed through their teens, the differences in P1 latency between the CI users and the normally hearing children increased. This is illustrated in Figure 8.13 where P1 latency is plotted as a function of (chronological) age for implanted children ranging from six to 17 years of age. These data are super-imposed on functions representing the mean P1 latency for normally hearing children ± 1 standard deviation (SD). In contrast to the prediction of the earlier study, the cortical AEPs of the implanted children did not evolve a morphology similar to that of normally hearing teenagers or young adults. Rather, the cortical AEPs appeared to be locked in a state of immaturity, dominated by the P1 AEP and lacking the N1 peak that dominates the cortical AEPs of adults.

Based on the pattern of cortical AEP maturation that occurs in normally hearing children (Ponton et al., 2000a), the possibility exists that the immature AEP morphology of implanted children is related to the absence of a normal N1 peak. Modelling studies described by Ponton and Eggermont (2001), show that the large maturational changes in the auditory evoked potentials of normally hearing children occurring between the ages of five and 19 years of age can be almost entirely accounted for by an age-related increase in the N1 AEPs. Further justification for this model of maturation arises from patterns of neuro-anatomical maturation observed in the post-mortem examination of human auditory cortical tissue. Using an immuno-stain for axonal neurofilaments, Moore et al. (1997) showed that the axonal structure of deeper cortical layers up to the lower portions of layer III (as well as layer I) matured much earlier than upper layer III and II. While axonal neurofilament is apparent in these upper layers by five years of age, it still lacks the strong horizontal and vertical lattice-like structure that becomes characteristic by about 12 years of age. As argued by Steinschneider et al. (1994) and others, the N1 AEP likely reflects activation in upper layer III and II of the auditory cortex. It would therefore appear that the maturation of the

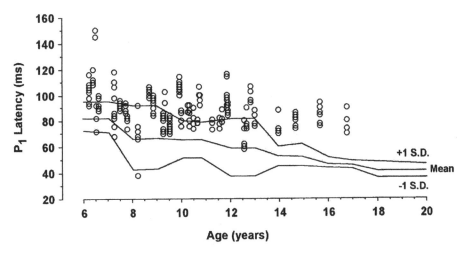

Figure 8.13. Longitudinal and cross-sectional P1 latency data (open circles) from CI children plotted as a function of age. These data are superimposed on functions representing the mean P1 latency ± 1 standard deviation (SD) for normally hearing children.

N1 potential in normally hearing children coincides with the emergence of a mature axonal structure in superficial layers of the auditory cortex. It is important to note that all of the deaf children included in this study had been implanted at least by seven years of age. Therefore, the absence of a normal N1 potential cannot be attributed to the absence of CI-driven input during this time period. Rather it appears that the absence of this AEP is related to an early period of auditory deprivation due to profound deafness prior to four or five years of age.

Application of cortical AEPs in training and rehabilitation programmes

Results of our research with CI users have shown that the cortical AEPs, including the MMN, are sensitive to both temporal differences (duration contrasts) and frequency differences (stimulation of different electrode pairs along the implant array). Examples are shown in Ponton and Don (1995). These findings raise the possibility that the MMN might be used to structure and monitor training and rehabilitation programmes in adults who show little benefit in speech recognition using their CI. Previous studies have suggested that a number of factors may affect spoken language recognition abilities with a cochlear implant, including access to a spectrally rich representation of the speech signal via the CI. One method of determining the extent to which a CI user has access to this information is to assess electrode discrimination. Poor electrode discrimination may reflect an impoverished and/or uneven distribution of surviving neural elements in the cochlea (Shannon, 1983; Busby and Clark, 2000).

We therefore initiated a pilot training study with an adult CI user focused on electrode discrimination. The individual selected to participate in this pilot project was a prelingually hearing-impaired, 36-year-old male who showed poor to moderate CI-assisted speech recognition abilities and poor electrode discrimination performance. His bilateral hearing loss was identified at 18 months of age and progressed to profound by age 29. At the onset of training, he had used a Nucleus CI22M implant for more than four years. Pretraining measures of consonant and vowel identification were 34% and 56%, respectively.

At the outset of the training programme, a complete psychophysical evaluation of the subject's electrode discrimination abilities was performed. We then recorded AEPs using electrode pair contrasts to evoke the MMN. The rationale behind the collection of the MMN data was to identify electrode pair contrasts that showed discrepant behavioural and neurophysiological discrimination results. Based on our studies of duration discrimination (Trautwein et al., 1998), we had shown that it was possible to obtain statistically significant MMN responses in the absence of behavioural discrimination. Presumably, this finding indicates that there can be preperceptual discrimination of auditory events in the cortex (as per the definition of the MMN), that is not always accessed at the perceptual level of cognitive processing. Thus, we collected MMN data for electrode pair contrasts that the subject discriminated easily and for contrasts that the subject could not discriminate.

A comparison of the psychophysical and electrophysiological data revealed discrepant discrimination results at a number of electrode locations. Four electrode contrasts where the MMN was present and behavioural discrimination was absent were identified and selected for training. A moderately intensive training programme was then initiated, which consisted of alternate sessions of discrimination training (testing with immediate feedback) and performance evaluation (testing without feedback). Training and evaluation were performed on a daily basis, two to three hours per day, five days per week, lasting a period of three weeks, focusing on two pairs of electrode contrasts at a time. At the end of the three-week training interval, the subject showed clear improvements in electrode discrimination for the trained contrasts. Perhaps more importantly, the results appeared to generalize, with improved discrimination performance observed for many non-trained contrasts. The signal detection measure of d' was applied as an index of improvement for the psychophysical data obtained using a three-interval forced choice task (with the first interval containing the reference). The average d' value for all electrode pair contrasts improved significantly from a pretraining value of 0.87 to a post-training value of 1.35 measured two weeks after the completion of training. While speech recognition training was not performed during the course of this study, the subject's speech recognition ability was routinely tested. Despite the absence of training, consonant and vowel identification improved from pretraining levels of 34% and 56%, respectively, to 51% and 63% respectively, at the completion of training.

These findings must be regarded as preliminary, but the results of this single-subject study suggest that neurophysiological responses such as the MMN may be used to both guide training and monitor a CI user's progress on an individual basis. Statistical analysis of the data showed moderate to strong correlations between psychophysical measures of discrimination (d') and MMN amplitude. Consequently, it may be possible to use this neurophysiological response to predict performance, or perhaps more importantly, predict the potential for performance.

An adult with good communication skills can provide rapid and accurate feedback in training situations. Therefore, the role of AEPs like the MMN to guide the selection of stimulus parameters for training may be redundant. However, neurophysiological data may still fulfil a role of monitoring the progress of training. Studies in non-human mammals (Takeuchi et al., 2000) and in humans (Tremblay et al., 1997; 1998; Menning et al., 2000) have demonstrated that training-related changes in the cortical AEPs emerge before behavioural changes become apparent. The obvious population that would benefit most from a reliable, objective, and passively recordable measure of auditory discrimination is young children. Confirmation of the preliminary findings of this study would be of significant value for training programmes focused on young implanted children who may have little or no experience with sound, and limited language and communication skills.

Conclusions

To date, the application of cortical AEPs with cochlear implant populations has been quite limited. Partly, this reflects the difficulty of reliably obtaining good quality AEPs that are not contaminated by stimulus artefact. Since the artefact is present from at least stimulus onset to offset, the AEP activity of interest may be entirely compromised for the duration of the stimulus. The use of short duration stimuli has the advantage of isolating the stimulus artefact away from the AEP of interest; but the presence of the artefact for the duration of the stimulus precludes recording AEPs elicited by realistic duration (100 to 500 ms) speech segments such as consonant–vowels (CVs). As shown by Kraus et al. (1993), it is possible to record speech evoked cortical AEPs in cochlear implant users, but it is unusual to reliably record them artefact free. If the cortical AEPs are recorded from a sufficiently large number of electrodes distributed across the scalp, it may be possible to identify a few channels that are uncontaminated or minimally contaminated by stimulus artefact. Application of advanced signal processing techniques such as independent components analysis to isolate and extract the prolonged stimulus artefact associated with speech segments and full words offers the possibility of recovering the AEPs at all electrode locations, even those adjacent to the implant hardware.

Use of the ICA technique provides the opportunity to study the cortical AEPs evoked by longer duration speech segments and words. At present this technique is available on a very limited number of commercial evoked potential systems. While speech evoked cortical potentials provide the most direct and easily interpretable information about speech-related processing in the cortex, many other directions of investigation with CI populations can be explored. Speech processing relies on a number of basic auditory processing skills that can be investigated neurophysiologically using short duration stimuli. For example, studies have shown that significant correlations exist between speech performance and basic psychophysical measures, such as electrode discrimination (Donaldson and Nelson, 2000), temporal modulation detection (Cazals et al., 1994), and gap detection (Cazals et al., 1991; Muchnik et al., 1993; Busby and Clark, 1999). Thus, AEP studies that focus on the frequency or temporal content of stimulation in CI users are worth consideration.

Studies of implanted children have expanded our knowledge of the effects that a period of auditory deprivation due to profound deafness has on the maturing human brain. The absence of sensory input appears to arrest maturation of at least some auditory cortical processes reflected in the AEPs. On the other hand, CI-driven stimulation of the central auditory system seems sufficient to restore at least some aspects of auditory maturation. This restoration of maturational process may however be limited by a critical period.

The data that we have collected from implanted children (as well as a large data set recorded by Sharma et al., personal communication) indicate that an early period of profound deafness permanently alters the cortical AEP morphology resulting in an absence of a normal N1 peak. This absence cannot be attributed to factors such as unilateral stimulation of the maturing central auditory system. In a parallel set of control studies, we have recorded cortical AEPs from children and teenagers with congenital profound unilateral deafness. The AEPs recorded from this group have a morphology similar to that of normally hearing children, containing a robust N1 potential. It therefore appears that a period of profound bilateral deafness that occurs in early childhood (prior to age five years) has a critical impact on cortical activity reflected in the N1, even though this AEP does not emerge until later in childhood (except at very slow stimulus presentation rates). As mentioned in a previous section, the spoken language processing skills of the implanted children included in these studies all benefited from use of the CI. Therefore, the neural processes generating N1 do not seem particularly critical to spoken language processing. Rather these results indicate that the functional significance of the N1 as a measure of the conscious detection of an auditory event (Hyde, 1997) has to be reconsidered.

As with any other clinical or research application using AEPs, success or failure is largely determined by methodological factors. Proper subject preparation, including careful electrode application, is a critical factor affecting the quality of the recorded AEP data. The quality of the AEPs is strongly affected by the recording environment. It is also important to ensure sufficient data is collected so that interpretation reflects the characteristics of the AEPs and not the background noise containing the AEPs. Many methodological shortcuts have been described for recording cortical AEPs, including the MMN. However, it is important to ensure that these shortcuts do not compromise the integrity of the AEPs or jeopardize the ability to interpret the data once it is recorded. Finally, when objective methods of AEP detection are available they should be applied.

Preliminary studies suggest a clinical application of cortical AEPs in guiding and monitoring behavioural training. The development of cortical AEP-assisted training programmes has its greatest potential application with implanted children. However, considerable work is needed to verify this application and to optimize it for use with young children.

References

Abbas PJ, Brown CJ, Shallop JK, Firszt JB, Hughes ML, Hong SH, Staller SJ (1999) Summary of results using the Nucleus CI24M implant to record the electrically evoked compound action potential. Ear Hear 20: 45–59.

Alho K (1995) Cerebral generators of mismatch negativity (MMN) and its magnetic counterpart (MMNm) elicited by sound changes. Ear Hear 16: 38–50.

Bell AJ, Sejnowski TJ (1995) An information-maximization approach to blind separation and blind deconvolution. Neural Comput 7: 1129–59.

Buchwald JS, Rubenstein EH, Schwafel J, Strandburg RJ (1991) Midlatency auditory evoked responses: differential effects of a cholinergic agonist and antagonist. Electroencephalogr Clin Neurophysiol 80: 303–9.

Busby PA, Clark GM (1999) Gap detection by early-deafened cochlear-implant subjects. J Acoust Soc Am 105: 1841–52.

Busby PA, Clark GM (2000) Pitch estimation by early-deafened subjects using a multiple-electrode cochlear implant. J Acoust Soc Am 107: 547–58.

Cacace AT, Satya-Murti S, Wolpaw JR (1990) Human middle-latency auditory evoked potentials: vertex and temporal components. Electroencephalogr Clin Neurophysiol 77: 6–18.

Cazals Y, Pelizzone M, Kasper A, Montandon P (1991) Indication of a relation between speech perception and temporal resolution for cochlear implantees. Ann Otol Rhinol Laryngol 100: 893–5.

Cazals Y, Pelizzone M, Saudan O, Boex C (1994) Low-pass filtering in amplitude modulation detection associated with vowel and consonant identification in subjects with cochlear implants. J Acoust Soc Am 96: 2048–54.

Cheour M, Ceponien R, Lehtokoski A, Luuk A, Allik J, Alho K, Näätänen R (1998) Development of language-specific phoneme representations in the infant brain. Nature Neuroscience 1: 351–3.

Creutzfeldt OD, Watanabe S, Lux HD (1966) Relations between EEG phenomena and potentials of single cortical cells. I. Evoked responses after thalamic and epicortical stimulation. Electroencephalogr Clin Neurophysiol 20: 1–18.

Dehaene-Lambertz G (1997) Electrophysiological correlates of categorical phoneme perception in adults. NeuroReport 8: 919–24.

Don M, Elberling C, Waring MD (1984) Objective detection of averaged auditory brainstem responses. Scand Audiol 13: 219–28.

Donaldson GS, Nelson DA (2000) Place-pitch sensitivity and its relation to consonant recognition by cochlear implant listeners using the MPEAK and SPEAK speech processing strategies. J Acoust Soc Am 107: 1645–58.

Edgington ES (1995) Randomization Tests. New York: Decker.

Elberling C, Don M (1984) Quality estimation of averaged auditory brainstem responses. Scand Audiol 13: 187–97.

Erwin RJ, Buchwald JS (1986a) Midlatency auditory evoked responses: differential recovery cycle characteristics. Electroencephalogr Clin Neurophysiol 64: 417–23.

Erwin RJ, Buchwald JS (1986b) Midlatency auditory evoked responses: differential effects of sleep in humans. Electroencephalogr Clin Neurophysiol 65: 383–92.

Fischer C, Bognar L, Turjman F, Lapras C (1995) Auditory evoked potentials in a patient with a unilateral lesion of the inferior colliculus and medial geniculate body. Electroencephalogr Clin Neurophysiol 96: 261–7.

Giard M-H, Perrin F, Echallier JF, Thevenet M, Froment JC, Pernier J (1994) Dissociation of temporal and frontal components in the human auditory N1 wave: a scalp current density and dipole model analysis. Electroencephalogr Clin Neurophysiol 92: 238–52.

Giard M-H, Perrin F, Pernier J, Bouchet P (1990) Brain generators implicated in processing auditory stimulus deviance: a topographic event-related potential study. Psychophysiology 27: 627–40.

Graybiel AM (1973) The thalamo-cortical projection of the so-called posterior nuclear group: a study with anterograde degeneration methods in the cat. Brain Res 49: 229–44.

Guthrie D, Buchwald JS (1991) Significance testing of difference potentials. Psychophysiology 28: 240–4.

Hari R, Pelizzone M, Mäkelä J, Hällström J, Huttenen J, Knuutila J (1988) Neuromagnetic responses from a deaf subject to stimuli presented through a multi-channel cochlear prosthesis. Ear Hear 9: 148–52.

Hyde M (1997) The N1 response and its applications. Audiol Neurootol 2: 281–307.

Hyvärinen A, Oja E (2000) Independent component analysis: algorithms and applications. Neural Networks 13: 411–30.

Jacobson GP (1994) Magnetoencephalographic studies of auditory system function. J Clin Neurophysiol 11: 343–64.

Jasper HH (1958) The ten-twenty system of the International Federation. Electroencephalogr Clin Neurophysiol 10: 371-5.

Jutten C, Herault J (1991) Blind separation of sources, part I: An adaptive algorithm based on neuromimetic architecture. Signal Processing 24: 1-10.

Kaas JH, Hackett TA (2000) Subdivisions of auditory cortex and processing streams in primates. Proc Natl Acad Sci USA 97: 11793-9.

Kandel ER, Schwartz JH, Jessell TM (1991) Principals of Neural Science. New York: Elsevier.

Knight RT, Hillyard SA, Woods DL, Neville HJ (1980) The effects of frontal and temporal-parietal lesions on the auditory evoked potentials. Electroencephalogr Clin Neurophysiol 50: 112-24.

Kraus N, McGee T (1993) Clinical implications of primary and nonprimary pathway contributions to the middle latency response generating system. Ear Hear 14: 36-48.

Kraus N, McGee TJ, Carrell TD, Zecker SG, Nicol TG, Koch DB (1996) Auditory neurophysiologic responses and discrimination deficits in children with learning problems. Science 273: 971-3.

Kraus N, McGee T, Littman T, Nicol T, King C (1994) Nonprimary auditory thalamic representation of acoustic change. J Neurophysiol 72: 1270-7.

Kraus N, Micco AG, Koch DB, McGee T, Carrell T, Wiet R, Weingarten C, Sharma A (1993) The mismatch negativity cortical evoked potential elicited by speech in cochlear implant users. Hear Res 65: 118-24.

Lennartz RC, Weinberger NM (1992) Frequency-specific receptive field plasticity in the medial geniculate body induced by Pavlovian fear conditioning is expressed in the anesthetized brain. Behav Neurosci 106: 484-97.

Liëgeois-Chauvel C, Musolino A, Badier JM, Marquis P, Chauvel P (1994) Evoked potentials recorded from the auditory cortex in man: evaluation and topography of the middle latency components. Electroencephalogr Clin Neurophysiol 92: 204-14.

Makeig S, Bell AJ, Jung T-P, Sejnowski TJ (1996) Independent components analysis of electroencephalographic data. Advanced Neural Information Processing Systems 8: 145-51.

Makeig S, Jung T-P, Bell AJ, Ghahremani D, Sejnowski TJ (1997) Blind separation of event-related brain responses into independent components. Proc Natl Acad Sci U S A 94: 10979-84.

Makeig S, Westerfield M, Jung T-P, Covington J, Townsend J, Sejnowski TJ, Courchesne E (1999a) Independent components of the late positive response complex in a visual spatial attention task. J Neurosci 19: 2665-80.

Makeig S, Westerfield M, Townsend J, Jung T-P, Courchesne E, Sejnowski TJ (1999b) Independent components of the early event-related potential in a visual spatial attention task. Philos Trans Biol Sci 354: 1135-44.

Mäkelä JP, Hämäläinen M, Hari R, McEvoy L (1994) Whole-head mapping of middle-latency auditory evoked magnetic fields. Electroencephalogr Clin Neurophysiol 92: 414-21.

Mäkelä JP, Hari R (1992) Neuromagnetic auditory evoked responses after a stroke in the right temporal lobe. Neuroreport 3: 94-6.

Mäkelä JP, McEvoy L (1996) Auditory evoked fields to illusory sound source movements. Exp Brain Res 110: 446-54.

Mann V, Soli SD (1991) Perceptual order and the effect of vocalic context of fricative perception. Perception and Psychophysics 49: 399-411.

McCandlish CA, Li CX, Waters RS, Howard EM (1996) Digit removal leads to discrepancies between the structural and functional organization of the forepaw barrel subfield in layer IV of rat primary somatosensory cortex. Exp Brain Res 108:417-26.

Menning H, Roberts LE, Pantev C (2000) Plastic changes in the auditory cortex induced by intensive frequency discrimination training. Neuroreport 11: 817-22.

Miztdorf U (1986) The physiological causes of VEP: Current source density analysis of electrically and visually evoked potentials. In Cracco RQ, Bodis-Wollner I, Alan R (eds) Evoked Potentials. New York: Liss Inc, pp. 141-54.

Moore JK, Guan Y-L, Wu BJ-C (1997) Maturation of human auditory cortex: laminar cytoarchitecture and axonal ingrowth. Association for Research in Otolaryngology Abstracts 109: 98.

Møller AR, Jannetta PJ (1982) Auditory evoked potentials recorded intracranially from the brainstem in man. Exp Neurol 78: 144-57.

Muchnik, C, Taitelbaum, R, Tene S, Hildesheimer M (1993) Auditory temporal resolution and open speech recognition in cochlear implant recipients. Scand Audiol 23: 105-9.

Näätänen R (1990) The role of attention in auditory information processing as revealed by event-related potentials and other brain measures of cognitive function. Behav Brain Sci 13: 201-88.

Näätänen R (2001) The perception of speech sound by the human brain as reflected by the mismatch negativity (MMN) and its magnetic equivalent (MMNm). Psychophysiology 38: 1-21.

Näätänen R, Lehtokoski A, Lennes M, Cheour M, Huotilainen M, Iivonen A, Valnio M, Alku P, Iilmoniemi RJ, Luuk A, Allik J, Sinkkonen J, Alho K (1997) Language-specific phoneme representations revealed by electric and magnetic brain responses. Nature 385: 432-4.

Näätänen R, Michie P (1979) Early selective attention effects on the evoked potential. A critical review and reinterpretation. Biol Psychol 8: 81-136.

Näätänen R, Picton TW (1987) The N1 wave of the human electric and magnetic response to sound: a review and analysis of the component structure. Psychophysiology 24: 375-425.

Pelizzone M, Hari R, Mäkelä J, Kaukoranta E, Montandon P (1986) Activation of the auditory cortex by cochlear stimulation in a deaf patient. Neurosci Lett 68: 192-6.

Pelizzone M, Hari R, Mäkelä J, Kauloranta E, Montandon P (1987) Cortical activity evoked by a multi-channel cochlear prosthesis. Acta Otolaryngol 103: 632-6.

Pelizzone M, Kasper A, Hari R, Karhu J, Montandon P (1991) Bilateral electrical stimulation of a congenitally-deaf ear and of an acquired-deaf ear. Acta Otolaryngol 111: 263-8.

Ponton CW, Don M (1995) The mismatch negativity in cochlear implant users. Ear Hear 16: 131-46.

Ponton CW, Eggermont JJ (2001) Of kittens and kids: altered cortical maturation following profound deafness and cochlear implant use. Audiol Neurootol 6: 263-80.

Ponton CW, Don M, Eggermont JJ, Kwong B (1997) Integrated MMN (MMNi): a noise free representation that allows distribution free single-point statistical tests. Electroencephalogr Clin Neurophysiol 104: 143-50.

Ponton CW, Don M, Eggermont JJ, Waring MD, Kwong B, Cunningham J, Trautwein P (2000a) Maturation of the mismatch negativity: Effects of profound deafness and cochlear implant use. Audiol Neurootol 5: 167-85.

Ponton CW, Don M, Eggermont JJ, Waring MD, Kwong B, Masuda A (1996a) Auditory system plasticity in children after long periods of complete deafness. Neuroreport 8: 61–5.

Ponton CW, Don M, Eggermont JJ, Waring MD, Masuda A (1996b) Maturation of human cortical auditory function: differences between normal hearing and cochlear implant children. Ear Hear 17: 430–7.

Ponton CW, Don M, Waring MD, Eggermont JJ, Masuda A (1993) Spatio-temporal modeling of evoked potentials to acoustic and cochlear implant stimulation. Electroencephalogr Clin Neurophysiol, 88: 478–93.

Ponton CW, Eggermont JJ, Don M, Kwong B (2000b) Maturation of human central auditory system activity: Evidence from multi-channel evoked potentials. Clin Neurophysiol 111: 220–36.

Ponton CW, Moore JK, Eggermont JJ (1999) Prolonged deafness limits auditory system developmental plasticity: evidence from an evoked potentials study in children with cochlear implants. Scand Audiol 28 (Suppl 51): 13–22.

Reite M, Teale P, Zimmerman J, Davis K, Whalen J (1988) Source location of a 50 ms latency auditory evoked field component. Electroencephalogr Clin Neurophysiol 70: 490–8.

Rif J, Hari R, Hamalainen MS, Sams M (1991) Auditory attention affects two different areas in the human supratemporal cortex. Electroencephalogr Clin Neurophysiol 79: 464–72.

Ritter W, Deacon, D, Gomes H, Javitt DC, Vaughan HG (1995) The mismatch negativity of event-related potentials as a probe of transient auditory memory: a review. Ear Hear 16: 52–67.

Scherg M (1990) Fundamentals of dipole source analysis. In Grandori F, Hoke M, Romani GL (eds) Auditory Evoked Magnetic Fields and Electric Potentials. Basel: Karger, pp. 40–69.

Scherg M, Vasjar J, Picton TW (1989) A source analysis of the late human auditory evoked potentials. J Cognitive Neurosci 1: 336–55.

Scherg M, Von Cramon D (1986) Evoked dipole source potentials of the human auditory cortex. Electroencephalogr Clin Neurophysiol 65: 344–60.

Shannon RV (1983) Multichannel electrical stimulation of the auditory nerve in man. II. Channel interaction. Hear Res 12(1): 1–16.

Shannon RV, Adams DD, Ferrel RL, Palumbo RL, Grandgenett M (1990) A computer interface for psychophysical and speech research with the Nucleus cochlear implant. J Acoust Soc Am 87: 905–7.

Sharma A, Dorman MF (2000) Neurophysiologic correlates of cross-language phonetic perception. J Acoust Soc Am 107: 2697–703.

Sharma A, Kraus N, McGee T, Carrell T, Nicol T (1993) Acoustic versus phonetic representation of speech as reflected by the mismatch negativity event-related potential. Electroencephalogr Clin Neurophysiol 88: 64–71.

Skinner JE, Yingling CD (1977) Central gating mechanisms that regulate event-related potentials and behavior: a neural model for attention. In: Desmedt JE (ed.) Attention, Voluntary Contraction and Event-Related Cerebral Potentials. Progress in Clinical Neurophysiology. Basel: Karger, pp. 30–69.

Steinschneider M, Schroeder CE, Arezzo JC, Vaughan Jr HG (1994) Speech-evoked activity in primary auditory cortex: effects of voice onset time. Electroencephalogr Clin Neurophysiol 92: 30–43.

Takeuchi S, Jodo E, Suzuki Y, Matsuki T, Hoshino KY, Niwa SI, Kayama Y (2000) ERP development in the rat in the course of learning two-tone discrimination task. Neuroreport 11: 333-6.

Tonnquist-Uhlén I (1996) Topography of auditory evoked cortical potentials in children with severe language impairment. Scand Audiol 25 (Suppl. 44): 1-40.

Tonnquist-Uhlén I, Ponton CW, Eggermont JJ, Kwong B, Don M (in press) Maturation of the central auditory system activity: The T-complex. Clin Neurophysiol.

Trautwein PG, Ponton CW, Kwong B, Waring MD (1998) Neurophysiological and psychophysical measures of duration discrimination in normal-hearing adults and adults with cochlear implants. Proc 16th Int Congr Acoust and 135th Meeting Ac Soc Am, pp. 877-8.

Tremblay K, Kraus N, Carrell TD, McGee T (1997) Central auditory system plasticity: generalization to novel stimuli following listening training. J Ac Soc Am 102: 3762-73.

Tremblay K, Kraus N, McGee T (1998) The time course of auditory perceptual learning: neurophysiological changes during speech-sound training. Neuroreport 9: 3557-60.

Vaughan H, Arezzo J (1988) The neural basis of event-related potentials. In Picton TW (ed.) Human Event-related Potentials. Amsterdam: Elsevier Science Publishers, pp. 45-96.

Weinberger NM (1993) Learning-induced changes of auditory receptive fields. Curr Opin Neurobiol 3: 570-7.

Weinberger NM, Diamond DM (1987) Physiological plasticity in auditory cortex: rapid induction by learning. Prog Neurobiol 29: 1-55.

Winer JA (1992) The functional architecture of the medial geniculate nucleus and the primary auditory cortex. In Webster DB, Popper AN, Fay RR (eds) The Mammalian Auditory Pathway: Neuroanatomy. New York: Springer-Verlag, pp. 222-409.

Winkler I, Lehtokoski A, Alku P, Vainio M, Czigler I, Csepe V, Aaltonen O, Raimo I, Alho K, Lang H, Iivonen A, Naatanen R (1999) Pre-attentive detection of vowel contrasts utilizes both phonetic and auditory memory representations. Brain Res Cogn Brain Res 7: 357-69.

Wolpaw JR, Penry JK (1975) A temporal component of the AEP. Electroencephalogr Clin Neurophysiol 39: 609-20.

Woods DL, Knight RT, Scabini D (1993) Anatomical substrates of auditory selective attention: behavioral and electrophysiological effects of posterior association cortex lesions. Cogn Brain Res 1: 227-40.

Yingling CD, Skinner JE (1977) Gating of thalamic input to cerebral cortex by nucleus reticularis laminaris. In Desmedt JE (ed.) Attention, Voluntary Contraction and Event-Related Cerebral Potentials. Progress in Clinical Neurophysiology. Basel: Karger, pp. 70-96.

Index

Printed and bound by CPI Group (UK) Ltd, Croydon, CR0 4YY

16/04/2025

14658512-0001